SEXUALLY TRANSMITTED INFECTIONS

MARY-CLAIRE MASON is a freelance journalist with a special interest in health. She is a member of the Medical Journalists' Association and the Guild of Health Writers. She has written for the national press, as well as for women's magazines such as *Bella*, *Woman's Realm* and *Essentials*. She is the author of *Coping with Fibroids* and co-author, with Dr Elaine Smith, of *Rheumatoid Arthritis: Your Medication Explained*, both published by Sheldon Press. She lives in London with her husband, two cats and a Dalmatian.

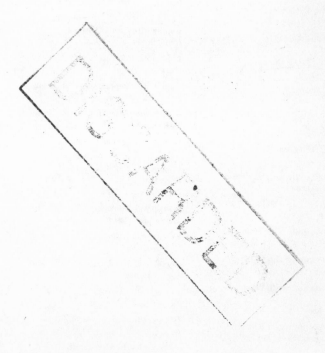

Overcoming Common Problems Series

For a full list of titles please contact
Sheldon Press, 1 Marylebone Road, London NW1 4DU

Overcoming Common Problems Series

7.32
m

Overcoming Common Problems Series

How to Stick to a Diet
Deborah Steinberg and Dr Windy Dryden

How to Stop Worrying
Dr Frank Tallis

The How to Study Book
Alan Brown

How to Succeed as a Single Parent
Carole Baldock

How to Untangle Your Emotional Knots
Dr Windy Dryden and Jack Gordon

How to Write a Successful CV
Joanna Gutmann

Hysterectomy
Suzie Hayman

The Irritable Bowel Diet Book
Rosemary Nicol

The Irritable Bowel Stress Book
Rosemary Nicol

Is HRT Right for You?
Dr Anne MacGregor

Jealousy
Dr Paul Hauck

Living with Asthma
Dr Robert Youngson

Living with Crohn's Disease
Dr Joan Gomez

Living with Diabetes
Dr Joan Gomez

Living with Fibromyalgia
Christine Craggs-Hinton

Living with Grief
Dr Tony Lake

Living with High Blood Pressure
Dr Tom Smith

Living with Nut Allergies
Karen Evennett

Living with Osteoporosis
Dr Joan Gomez

Living with a Stoma
Dr Craig White

Making Friends with Your Stepchildren
Rosemary Wells

Motor Neurone Disease – A Family Affair
Dr David Oliver

Overcoming Anger
Dr Windy Dryden

Overcoming Anxiety
Dr Windy Dryden

Overcoming Guilt
Dr Windy Dryden

Overcoming Jealousy
Dr Windy Dryden

Overcoming Procrastination
Dr Windy Dryden

Overcoming Shame
Dr Windy Dryden

Overcoming Your Addictions
Dr Windy Dryden and
Dr Walter Matweychuk

The Parkinson's Disease Handbook
Dr Richard Godwin-Austen

The PMS Diet Book
Karen Evennett

A Positive Thought for Every Day
Dr Windy Dryden

Rheumatoid Arthritis
Mary-Claire Mason and Dr Elaine Smith

Second Time Around
Anne Lovell

Serious Mental Illness – A Family Affair
Gwen Howe

Shift Your Thinking, Change Your Life
Mo Shapiro

The Stress Workbook
Joanna Gutmann

The Subfertility Handbook
Virginia Ironside and Sarah Biggs

Successful Au Pairs
Hilli Matthews

Talking with Confidence
Don Gabor

Ten Steps to Positive Living
Dr Windy Dryden

Think Your Way to Happiness
Dr Windy Dryden and Jack Gordon

The Travellers' Good Health Guide
Ted Lankester

Understanding Obsessions and Compulsions
Dr Frank Tallis

Understanding Sex and Relationships
Rosemary Stones

Understanding Your Personality
Patricia Hedges

Work–Life Balance
Gordon and Ronni Lamont

Sexually Transmitted Infections

What You Need To Know

Mary-Claire Mason

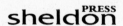

Published in Great Britain in 2002 by
Sheldon Press
1 Marylebone Road
London NW1 4DU

British Library Cataloguing-in-Publication Data
A catalogue record for this book is available from the British Library

ISBN 0–85969–868–8

Typeset by Deltatype Limited, Birkenhead, Merseyside
Printed in Great Britain by Biddles Ltd
www.biddles.co.uk

Contents

1

Why You Need to Know about Sexually Transmitted Infections

Sex involves such a mix of physical and emotional feelings that even if you're sexually experienced the risks involved in having sex can get pushed to one side. And if you've just started having sex it's easy to be so swept up with it all that you don't even think what risks you may be running.

An unwanted pregnancy is the risk that most people are aware of but what tends to get forgotten, overlooked or missed is the very real risk of picking up an infection as a result of sex. Twenty-year-old college student Susan's comment illustrates this: 'What people my age are most scared about is getting pregnant.'

My own experience is a good example of how risks from sexually transmitted infections (STIs) are not known about or ignored. STIs have always been around and when I was in my teens at school over 30 years ago I remember having some sort of lesson on venereal disease (VD), the name used for STIs in those days. I don't remember it in detail but the subject seemed shocking. AIDS wasn't on the agenda then and there was no mention of safer sex practices. If I remember correctly, we were told that it was men – particularly those who slept with prostitutes – who were most at risk from VD, and the message was that you shouldn't have sex before marriage and that was it. Though the 'lesson' was alarming it didn't seem to have anything to do with me, and I couldn't relate it to my own experience, so I didn't take the message on board.

In my late teens I was friends for a short time with a man who I suspected of having lots of other girlfriends who he slept with. We had sex just once and it was unprotected – that is, no condom was used – but that time came to haunt me years later when in my mid-twenties I was referred to a sexual health clinic because of a suspicious vaginal discharge.

After much anguish and uncertainty about my test results, I was assured finally that they were clear and that I didn't have anything wrong with me. But to this day I'm not certain what was behind that

1

discharge, and wonder if it could have been linked to that 'episode' in my late teens, even though at the time I was told that this wasn't possible.

The main point about my story is that I wish I'd known what risks I was taking when I slept with that man. Yes, I knew about the pregnancy one but I didn't think about anything else, or perhaps I pushed other thoughts to the back of my mind.

STIs – also called 'sexually transmitted diseases' – are a fact of life and have always been the downside of sex. Most people today know about one of them – HIV (the human immunodeficiency virus) which over time can seriously damage your immune system causing AIDS (acquired immune deficiency syndrome) – but what's less well known is that there are many other STIs, well over 15 in fact.

There was a lot of information about how to protect yourself against HIV, the life-threatening virus, in the early 1980s and, as a result of various campaigns, people started to practise safer sex and the numbers of cases of many other STIs started to fall in the late 1980s and early 1990s.

But that pattern has changed, perhaps because it's tempting to think that, with better understanding of HIV and developments in drug treatments, 'there isn't a problem out there' and that safer sex (or 'protected' sex – this is explained and discussed in Chapter 3) isn't necessary. The Durex Report 2001 mentioned in Chapter 3 reports that unprotected sex is on the increase.

But there *is* a problem 'out there'. In 1990 there were 624,269 infection cases at sexual health clinics but by 1999 this figure had risen to over one million.

Research figures show that there was a big increase in certain STIs between 1995 and 1999; for instance, by 76 per cent for chlamydia, 55 per cent for gonorrhoea – both STIs that can cause a lot of health problems and also infertility if not treated early on – as well as a 20 per cent increase for genital warts. The figures also show that you're most at risk of getting these sorts of STIs if you're under 25.

HIV cases are also on the increase. In 2000 there were 3,435 new HIV cases, 14 per cent higher than in 1999. Gay and bisexual men are still the people who are at most risk of getting infected with HIV, but in 1999 and 2000 the number of new cases of HIV in men having sex with women was higher than in men having sex with men.

As a result of these findings the first ever National Strategy for Sexual Health and HIV, published by the Department of Health in 2001, aims to prevent the spread of STIs through an information campaign as well as to improve services for people who need treatment.

This book covers what you need to know about a range of STIs, from potentially life-threatening ones such as HIV and syphilis, to common ones such as chlamydia, which are dangerous because they can cause so much damage if not treated early on. I've also included others that aren't serious as such but can cause a lot of misery, but I haven't included infections that are very rare in the United Kingdom such as donovanosis.

Something that people often aren't aware of but that is very important is the relationship between STIs and pregnancy so I've talked about this because sometimes there's a risk that an infection can be passed to your baby.

I've also looked at some commonly held myths about STIs and at where to go for the best help. It's important to get treatment if you suspect you could have an infection because many STIs can be cured with simple, highly effective treatment, and the sooner you get treatment the better, to help prevent the sorts of complications that can occur if infections aren't treated. It's a point I keep repeating because it's so important.

I've also talked about STIs such as herpes and looked at the issues that come up when you live with this infection, which can't be cured at the moment but which isn't usually a huge problem for most people.

Prevention has to be the key and as a result the whole of Chapter 3 is devoted to this. Prevention is not as easy as it sounds because it means practising 'safer sex' and in order to do this you need to be able to talk openly and honestly about sexual health issues with your partner.

This can be hugely difficult and embarrassing for many of us to do, even in well-established relationships let alone new ones. If you've just started having sex, you need to learn how to talk about these issues on top of all the other things you may be struggling with. But it's really important to develop safer sex skills because in the end your sex life will be the better for being able to talk about sex and all the issues that go with it, and you'll be safeguarding your health.

2

An Introduction to Sexually Transmitted Infections

What are sexually transmitted infections?

Sexually transmitted infections (STIs) are infections that are spread through sexual contact. But it's not quite as simple as this because infections such as HIV and hepatitis B can also be spread in other ways; for instance, through infected blood from transfusions, when sharing drug-injecting equipment or by other things that pierce the skin, such as tattooing and body-piercing. Others, such as bacterial vaginosis and thrush aren't strictly speaking STIs because you can get them without being sexually active. Many of the infections can also be passed by a pregnant mum to her baby.

What are STIs caused by?

Some STIs are spread by bacteria (e.g. chlamydia, gonorrhoea), others by viruses (e.g. HIV, herpes, hepatitis A, B, C and genital warts), and some by parasites (e.g. pubic lice and scabies).

How are they spread?

STIs are spread through vaginal fluid, semen or infected blood during sex but they're not necessarily all passed on in the same way. Infections such as chlamydia are passed on through vaginal, anal and oral sex – that is, the penis enters the vagina, anus or mouth – whereas others such as herpes and genital warts can be caught through skin-to-skin contact.

How many people get STIs?

Figures from the Public Health Laboratory Service (PHLS), which monitors the numbers of cases of STIs each year, show (as I said in Chapter 1) that there's been an increase in the numbers of certain STIs since 1995.

Before this, cases of many STIs had been falling or had at least remained unchanged and the PHLS wonders whether the decline in infections was due to people practising safer sex as a result of all the messages about safer sex and HIV in the 1980s.

But the picture has now changed. Here are figures in 1999 for some of the most common infections: for chlamydia: 24,311 infections in men and 32,544 in women; for gonorrhoea: 11,289 cases in men and 5,181 in women; and for a first attack of genital warts: 37,765 cases in men and 34,468 in women.

How serious are STIs and can they be cured?

Most STIs can be cured with simple treatment. The sooner they're treated the better because the longer they're in the body the greater the risk of complications. Chlamydia, for example, can result in serious problems if it's untreated, including infertility in both men and women (especially women). Untreated syphilis is very serious and eventually results in damage to the heart, brain and nervous system. Hepatitis B causes liver problems.

Some STIs, such as genital herpes and warts, can't be cured at the moment but don't generally cause problems. HIV can't be cured currently but drug treatments have improved the outlook for this life-threatening infection.

What are the symptoms?

Symptoms vary according to the specific STI and this is looked at in more detail in the later chapters. However, here are the most common sorts of warning signs and symptoms.

Women

It's normal to have some vaginal discharge because a slightly acidic fluid keeps the vagina moist, clean and healthy. The amount of discharge can vary for hormonal reasons; for instance, some women get a lot of slippery, egg-white-type discharge around the time of ovulation each month when an egg is released.

But the discharge is likely to be abnormal and could be a sign of an STI if, for instance, it smells, itches, irritates, changes colour or is blood-stained.

Men

There may be a discharge from the penis and discomfort and pain around the testicles and in the groin.

Both sexes

Other symptoms that can affect both men and women include pain when peeing or more frequent urination, or itching, sores, blisters in the genital area, rashes, painful sex, discharge from the anus.

No symptoms

Don't assume that if you have no symptoms you're free of infection. Some of the infections may not cause any symptoms early on or only at certain stages so you may not have any symptoms until months or years later.

   If you've had symptoms and they've gone away don't assume you're better – if you've got an infection you need treatment even if you have no symptoms (see p. 10, 'When to get checked out' and 'Getting help', for what to do).

What about complications?

Complications can occur if the infection isn't treated.

Pelvic inflammatory disease

Pelvic inflammatory disease (PID), for instance, can occur if infections such as chlamydia or gonorrhoea aren't treated. PID is thought to occur in about 30 per cent of untreated infections.

   Procedures such as termination of pregnancy or fitting an intrauterine contraceptive device (IUD) can allow infections to travel up into the sterile pelvic cavity, which is why it's so important that checks are done, for example, before you have an IUD fitted.

   I've talked about IUDs at the end of this chapter but I'll mention them here as well because the point is so important. You should be asked about your sexual behaviour before an IUD is fitted: it's fine if you're in a stable relationship and both faithful to each other but it won't be recommended if you're at risk of getting an STI; for example, you're changing partners a lot and don't practise safer sex. If you're going to have an IUD, most doctors also think it's a good idea that you are tested for STIs before having one fitted in case you do have an infection.

PID happens when infections get into the pelvic cavity through the neck of the womb called 'the cervix' and affect the womb, ovaries and Fallopian tubes. An infection can be sudden and acute, causing symptoms such as severe abdominal pain, a high temperature, nausea, painful sex and vaginal discharge.

Chronic PID, which is defined as going on for over one month, can cause constant abdominal discomfort, very heavy and painful periods, tiredness and bleeding in between periods. However, *sometimes there are no symptoms with PID.*

In some women, PID can result in scarring of the Fallopian tubes, which results in infertility because the egg can't travel down the tube. Sometimes the pregnancy develops in the tube as an ectopic pregnancy which is a potentially life-threatening condition.

Diagnosis of PID is done by examining the pelvis, sometimes doing an ultrasound scan and doing a laparoscopy where a small tube is inserted into the abdomen so that the doctor can see what's going on inside the pelvis. Treatment is with a combination of antibiotics.

Epididymitis and prostatitis

Problems for men include epididymitis, which is inflammation of the epididymis – a coiled collecting tube attached to the top of the testicle where sperm are stored. The result is swollen painful testicles, and infertility can result if the epididymis becomes scarred and sperm get stuck inside it.

The prostate can become inflamed (prostatitis) if it's infected with bacteria such as chlamydia, and acute infections can produce problems such as fever and difficulty in urinating.

Treatment for epididymitis and prostatitis is with a combination of antibiotics.

Reiter's syndrome

Reiter's syndrome can develop in men and w
common in men. Symptoms may include pro
(the tube through which urine is excreted from
joint inflammation. Treatment is with anti-inflamma

Cervical cancer

There's a possible link to cervical cancer from genital warts
are caused by certain strains of the human papilloma virus (HP
which there are many. HPV is linked to cervical cancer but
strains involved are different from the ones normally associated with
genital warts so the risk is very small.

HIV

You may have a greater risk of catching HIV if you have or have
had other STIs. There are a couple of reasons for this. First, if you
have an STI you may have sores or cuts in the genital area, which
make it easier for HIV to be transmitted. Second, your immune
system – which defends you against infections – may have been
weakened by the presence of these other infections, which makes it
less able to protect you against HIV.

Fertility problems

Some infections may affect not only your fertility and your future
chances of getting pregnant, but also pregnancy itself – e.g.
increasing the likelihood of miscarriage, sometimes making the birth
more complicated as well as causing problems such as eye
infections, and lumps in the throat or genitals of the baby.

If there's any possibility that you're pregnant it's important to tell
the doctor treating you at the sexual health clinic as this may affect
the choice of drug given to you. Some drugs aren't so safe to use in
pregnancy because they might harm the developing baby.

If you or your partner has herpes also tell the midwife or doctor
who is helping you with your pregnancy (see the section on herpes
in Chapter 4).

ing an STI?

age, or sex, or whether
 get an infection.
ose who:

d particularly if under

ar or have had several

rtain infections, for
V whereas lesbians
...apter 3 for points about gay
...ation from the PHLS in mid-2001 said that
... women, gay and bisexual men are most vulnerable to STIs.

Susan, who I mentioned in Chapter 1, explains her understanding of the issues:

> Anyone is at risk, I guess, but you're more likely to have a problem if you sleep around, have a lot of casual sex and don't ever take precautions, though I suppose you could also have problems with someone who you thought was safe.

When to get checked out

It's a good idea to go to a clinic if you think you might have an infection because you've got suspicious signs or symptoms, or because you've had some risky sex (discussed in Chapter 3), or you and your partner want the 'all clear' before having unprotected sex i.e. not using condoms.

Getting help

The sexual health clinic

Sexual health clinics – or 'genito-urinary medicine (GUM) clinics' as they're called sometimes – are the best place to go for advice and help because the doctors, nurses and health advisers who run these clinics specialize in treating STIs and they're one-stop clinics, i.e.

clinics in which all tests and treatments are provided. (GPs may provide some tests and treatments but they're not usually specialists in STIs.)

What to expect from a clinic

- *Confidentiality*: you can expect your details to be kept private and treated confidentially – this is guaranteed by law – and you'll be given a number to identify you by. All of which means you don't need to worry about other people such as your GP being told about your visit unless of course you want them to know.
- *Understanding staff*: the thought of talking to a stranger about intimate details can be very frightening but it's important to give staff as much information as possible. Remember that they're trained and used to dealing with sexual health issues and will understand the sorts of worries and anxieties that you may have. They should help to put you at your ease.
- *Symptom check*: you don't need to have symptoms to be seen at a clinic.
- *Referrals*: you don't need to be referred to a clinic by your GP.
- *No Cost*: the service is free.
- *Help*: clinics are organized along the same lines though there may be some variations between them. They all have the same job of helping you. In addition to medical services, some also provide services such as counselling. So find out exactly what they can do for you. If you're gay, lesbian or bisexual ask if there are any special services for you as some clinics offer them; or ring the London Lesbian and Gay Switchboard for information (details in Chapter 8).
- *Segregation*: it's usual for men to be seen in one clinic and women in another. There may be separate waiting areas for men and women, though some clinics have a joint waiting area.
- *Waiting*: clinics are under a lot of pressure. Over one million people were seen at GUM clinics in 1999 – twice the number of people seen at the start of the 1990s – so clinics are very busy and may be overloaded at times. However, when you ring, make sure to say if you're in a lot of discomfort, in which case staff will try to fit you in as soon as possible. Meanwhile, find out if there's just one clinic in your area or several, because you may find that one

can fit you in sooner than the others. You don't have to live near a clinic to use it.

- *Walk-in service*: many clinics offer an appointment service and some a walk-in service though you may have to wait several hours to be seen at a walk-in clinic if it's very busy.
- *Treatment of all age groups*: clinics treat all age groups but Brook Advisory Centres offer clinics specially for young people – see Chapter 8 for more details.
- *Appointment times*: allow at least a couple of hours for your appointment – for diagnostic tests, results and treatment advice.

Clinic visit checklist

When you ring the clinic ask what information you need to take along. Also ask about how near to the clinic appointment you can pee – infectious organisms get flushed out when you urinate and so are harder to detect. The clinic will advise you how near to the appointment you can urinate – it's normally 3 hours.

Before you go along to the clinic, jot down a few things to help you in case your mind goes blank when you're asked questions. The sorts of things the clinic will want to know may include, for example:
- whether you have symptoms;
- what they are;
- when they started;
- date of your last period;
- why you think you might be at risk if you don't have symptoms;
- details about your sexual history, who you've slept with and the sort of sex you've had;
- whether you've had an STI before;
- whether you've been abroad recently and had sex with someone there (HIV is much more common in some other countries).

Let them know if you're on the contraceptive pill or if you've had an IUD fitted. Also give details about any medicines you're taking in case these affect any of the treatments you're given. Also mention whether you're allergic to any drugs. Give details about your last period, last smear test and whether you've had any unusual discharge or bleeding. Finally and most importantly tell the doctor if you're pregnant or think you could be.

If you've got your period, that won't interfere with tests (other than a cervical smear if that's needed for some reason) so there's no reason not to have the tests done if you've got your period unless you don't feel comfortable about having them done.

If you want to see a male or female doctor ask about this at your first appointment – clinics will try to help you on this one but it depends who they've got on their staff.

Examining you

During the examination, the doctor will look at the lymph nodes in your groin to see if they're swollen, and will want to have a look at the outside of your genitals and probably check your anus as well.

For women, the doctor may need to do an internal examination to see the inside of the vagina and the state of the cervix. You may feel worried about this, particularly if you've never had an internal examination before. The procedure shouldn't hurt but tell the doctor if you've never had one so they can take extra care to put you at your ease and make you feel comfortable.

You'll be asked to remove clothes below the waist and lie on the examination table with your knees bent. The doctor will gently press your abdomen to feel for anything that is unusual there. What's called a 'bimanual examination' may be done to check for pelvic swelling or tenderness. The doctor rests one hand on your abdomen just above the pubic bone while gently inserting one or two lubricated gloved fingers of their other hand into the vagina. By pushing upwards on the cervix and pressing down gently on the abdomen the doctor can check you inside.

An instrument called a 'speculum' is gently inserted into the vagina so that the doctor can check the inside of the vagina and the state of the cervix and take swabs.

In men the foreskin is pulled back so that the head of the penis can be examined, and the testicles are checked.

Diagnostic tests

Diagnostic blood and urine tests may be done and swabs taken from the genitals, anus and throat to check for infections like gonorrhoea. You may be tested for a range of STIs as it's possible to have more than one infection at a time. There's no one test for all infections.

Clinics have microscopes to do initial diagnostic tests, which means they can give some results quickly, but other tests have to be sent off to a laboratory and you may not get the results for a week or so.

The range of tests done depends on your history but a fairly standard set will look for: chlamydia, gonorrhoea, syphilis, thrush, herpes if you have sores, bacterial vaginosis and possibly hepatitis. You will not be tested for HIV without your knowledge or permission.

For women, specific tests include, for example, vaginal samples for thrush and bacterial vaginosis, a cervical swab for gonorrhoea, a urine sample for chlamydia, a blood test for syphilis. Swabs may also be taken from the throat and anus.

For men, swabs are taken using a cotton bud from the urethra (this may be slightly uncomfortable and may be a bit more painful if there's already some inflammation in the urethra) for infections such as gonorrhoea, a urine test for chlamydia, a blood test for syphilis. Swabs may also be taken from the throat and anus.

Staff will make sure you're having the test done at the right time because depending on the infection there's a period during which an infection may not show up. For example, it can take up to three months for enough antibodies to show up on an HIV test – so if you have the test done too soon after infection the results may come back negative.

Treatment

Here are some points to bear in mind.

- You may be treated 'just in case' – that is, as a precaution – for example, while waiting for test results or if there's any uncertainty about the results.
- Finish the treatment. Don't stop early because symptoms have gone and you think you're better. You need to finish the whole course of treatment.
- Discuss anything you don't understand with your clinic doctor or nurse, e.g. about your treatment and its side-effects, how long treatment lasts, whether the drugs interact with any other drugs you may be taking, whether there are any treatment options, what the cure rate is, and the chances of relapse.

- Sex isn't a good idea while you're being treated because of the risks of reinfection – you may well not want to have sex anyway if you feel uncomfortable or unwell, but as you start to feel better you may think it's safe to have sex. Don't! Get the clinic's advice on when you can safely start to have sex again. The situation is a bit different with STIs like herpes and genital warts, which can't be cured, in which case it's important to talk to the clinic about when and how you can safely have sex if you have one of these STIs.

- Partners – it's important that current and previous partners you've slept with know they could be carrying or at risk of having an infection, and it's important to remember that your present partner could reinfect you if they're infected and are not treated.

  You may feel very anxious about telling your partner that you have an infection and that they may be infected because of course this raises the question of where the infection came from in the first place. As we've already seen this isn't necessarily straightforward as infections can remain dormant in the body, sometimes for years, and you or your partner could have been infected at some time in the past without realizing it.

  Pick the right time to talk to your partner, preferably when there's plenty of time and you both feel reasonably relaxed. Explain that this is a joint problem that needs to be sorted out and that even if they don't have symptoms they should get checked out too.

  A health adviser at the clinic may be able to help prepare you for this discussion by identifying the sorts of issues that might arise, and how to talk about the subject using the right language rather than words that might just make matters worse and really upset your partner.

  If you feel you don't want to or can't talk to your partner, you can send them a contact slip or get one sent to them. The slip explains they may have an infection and should get checked out, but the slip won't reveal your identity.

- Tests are sometimes done to check if the treatment has worked and this needs to be done at the right time. For instance, with chlamydia, a test is not usually done until at least three weeks after finishing treatment, to avoid the risk of an inaccurate 'false positive' result; that is, the test may show you have an infection when in fact you don't, as bacteria that have been killed may still show up on the test.

Protecting yourself

Cervical smears

There's a possible link between some of the organisms that cause infections and cervical cancer. For example, a recent study suggested that chlamydia might be linked to this though this hasn't yet been proven. Meanwhile it makes sense to have regular cervical smears and not to ignore any possible warning signs, such as bleeding in between periods or after sex.

Contraceptive intrauterine devices

IUDs aren't a good idea unless you're in a stable relationship because there is a link between IUDs and STIs – sexual lifestyle. The IUD doesn't make you more likely to get an STI, but if you do get one the IUD may make it worse. This is because the IUD could make it easier for the infection to spread further and possibly cause problems such as pelvic inflammatory disease, which could result in infertility. Most doctors also recommend that before an IUD is fitted you're tested for STIs in case you've got an underlying infection, such as chlamydia, which can remain symptomless for several years and which could get pushed into the womb during insertion.

Summary

- Most STIs can be cured with simple drug treatment.
- It's better to get treated as soon as possible because untreated infections may cause serious health problems, including infertility.
- It's possible to have more than one infection at a time.

- Infections can be symptomless.
- If you've been successfully treated for an infection you can get it again if you have unsafe sex.
- Clinics provide all sorts of help. Some clinics also provide special information sessions for gays, lesbians and bisexuals. Brook Advisory Centres provide services for young people under 25.

3

How to Protect Yourself

This is the most important chapter in the book because it's all about safer sex or what is sometimes called 'safe sex', though no sex can be totally safe unless you're absolutely certain that you and your partner are infection-free. Unfortunately, this isn't a straightforward matter as you may not realize you have an STI and some infections can remain symptomless for weeks, months and even years.

Even someone who has never had sex before could be a possible source of infection, for example, if there is thrush or a herpes cold sore on the lip.

Safer sex can't guarantee that it is risk-free sex, and ideas about what it means in practice are changing as more is discovered about the various infections and how they're passed on. But what safer sex does do is to alert you to the possible risks you may be running and to let you know that there are steps you can take to protect yourself. Safer sex gives you choices.

When you first come across them, some of the safeguards may seem fussy, over the top and off-putting, apparently likely to take all the pleasure out of sex. You may be tempted to ditch the whole idea. Don't! The safer sex message is just pointing out that sex has risks attached to it and that you can take steps to reduce the risk and protect yourself. It's up to you to decide what level of risk is acceptable to you.

You may think that STIs aren't a real problem and that it's not worth bothering with safe sex. But all the research shows that people think this because they just don't know much about the real risks they're running and they believe infections happen only to other people. But safer sex practices are important and once you understand the general principles, safer sex will give you a sense of confidence and control and help you to protect your health now and in the future.

The second part of this chapter – which is equally important and which goes hand in hand with this section – is how to bring up the subject of safer sex and talk about it with your partner. It's not easy to talk about these things for all sorts of reasons that are looked at in the second part of the chapter, but by learning how to do this you'll be protecting your own and your partner's health and well-being.

What is safer sex?

When I asked what she thought safer sex meant, 20-year-old-Susan answered: 'It means using condoms, being careful about who you sleep with, knowing them properly, knowing something about their sexual history and knowing that you can trust them and that they'd tell you if they thought they had something.'

I think she gave a pretty good answer, but when it comes to the downside of sex Susan and her friends are very aware of the risks of an unwanted pregnancy but underplay the risks of picking up an infection. One of the reasons they do this is because they don't realize how many infections there are, how easily some can be caught and the potential seriousness of some of the infections.

Safer sex is all about cutting your chances of getting an infection. The only way to have virtually no risk is never to have had sex or any intimate body contact with anyone.

Safer sex means several things:

- *Understanding the sorts of risks you're running when you have sex.* For example, some forms of sexual activity are much more risky than others – unprotected (i.e. not using a condom) anal sex between gay men easily tops the list, particularly if you're the one being penetrated because tissue in the anus and rectum is more fragile and so more likely to get damaged, which makes it easier to get infected with HIV.
- *Realizing that some partners are more risky than others* (e.g. if you're a woman having unprotected sex with a bisexual man – the latest figures show bisexual men are more at risk of having infections) and the more partners you have the more risks you run.
- *Reducing your risk in various ways,* such as not sleeping with someone who you think is at high risk of having an infection or, if you do, using every possible way to protect yourself if you know absolutely nothing about the person (methods are listed below), or

19

you may decide that you need less protection with some people because you know a lot about their sexual history.

- *Understanding that penetrative sex is the most risky type of sex* (particularly for the person who is being penetrated) and especially with a new partner who you know nothing about. The best way of protecting yourself apart from not sleeping with the person is to have protected sex, that is, use a condom.

What do we know about STIs?

STIs are something many of us don't know much about. This ignorance is highlighted in a couple of points made in a new document already mentioned: the first National Strategy for Sexual Health and HIV produced by the Department of Health in 2001, which says:

- over a quarter of people in their mid-teens think that the contraceptive pill protects against infection – it doesn't.
- a 1999 study found that most people didn't know what chlamydia was yet it's one of the commonest STIs.

What's your risk?

Sexually active people of all ages – men and women, gay, straight and bisexual – can get infections but one point stands out: *younger people are more at risk*. A paper in 2000 from Brook, which provides a free confidential sex and contraceptive advisory service for young people, said that one in ten sexually active teenagers had an STI. And the Public Health Laboratory Service, while releasing early figures for STIs in 2000, says teenage women are at particular risk as well as gay and bisexual men. There's also an increase in all infections for the 35–44 age group.

The Durex Report 2001

More than 5,000 men and women between the ages of 16 and 55 were contacted for the Durex survey into sexual attitudes and behaviour in Britain. The results show that there's a lot of confusion about sexual safety when it comes to STIs and also that people are having sex at a younger age, which means they're more at risk. These are some of the findings:

- Three in ten people know someone who has had an STI and one in ten are aware of someone who has HIV.
- One in ten people admitted to having unprotected sex with a new partner in the last year – a figure which has more than doubled since 1994.
- People are having sex at a younger age (16- to 20-year-olds were 15 when they had first had sex, compared to 18 for the over-45s). In a Brook study some teenagers said they felt they'd had sex too soon.
- People are taking more risks, with 13 per cent saying they had unprotected sex with a new partner in the last year compared to 6 per cent in 1994.
- Younger people are taking more risks: 30 per cent of 16- to 20-year-olds had unprotected sex with a new partner in the last year compared with 7 per cent of the over-45s.
- People had unprotected sex for several reason. The largest group, 43 per cent, had used another contraceptive method (this means they were thinking about the pregnancy risks but not the infection risks), but 11 per cent said they weren't bothered about STIs and 24 per cent of 35- to 44-year-olds said they weren't worried about infections.
- People aged 25 to 34 had the most partners at an average of 10.6, compared to 9.9 for 21- to 24-year-olds and 6.2 for 16- to 20-year-olds.
- The survey revealed that although one in three people worried about getting infected with HIV, just four in 100 were concerned about getting other STIs.

What all this adds up to is that lots of us just don't know much about STIs, underestimate how serious some of them can be and think we could never be infected. And if you're in your teens you're likely to be so caught up with other issues when you start having sex that getting an infection is the last thing on your mind.

Sex – What's really risky?

This isn't a straightforward issue because, as we've seen, there are lots of STIs and they're not all passed on in the same way. But from what's known at the moment some sorts of sex are clearly more risky and some carry much less or hardly any risk.

High risk

Unprotected anal and vaginal sex is the riskiest sex to have if there's any possibility that your partner has one or more infections.

Some risk

With oral sex, the amount of risk will depend on which infections your partner has and also on whether you have gum disease or cuts and sores in the mouth or throat, which make it easier for some infections to be transmitted.

With HIV, information from the Public Health Laboratory Service says that the risk of getting HIV from oral sex is much smaller than from unprotected anal or vaginal sex, but that it's not risk-free and the risk could be higher than previously thought. Between 3 and 8 per cent of cases of HIV infection among men who have had sex with men may be due to oral sex.

Other STIs, such as gonorrhoea, syphilis, herpes and chlamydia, are more easily passed on through oral sex than HIV is.

Very low risk

These sorts of activities can be extremely pleasurable, exciting and satisfying for some people.

- Masturbating together without touching your partner's genitals.
- Mutual masturbation – it's possible that some infections (e.g. gonorrhoea) could be spread by touching your partner's genitals and then your own during mutual masturbation (but at the moment there's no known risk of getting HIV through mutual masturbation).
- Sex toys – if you use things like vibrators, clean them if you're sharing the toy or put a new condom on it between usages.

- Stroking, cuddling, hugging, fondling (without touching your partner's genitals).
- Kissing, provided neither of you has bleeding gums or cuts in the mouth or cold sores (cold sores carry the herpes virus) around the mouth. Love bites in theory could provide a way for viral infections to get into the body through broken skin but the amount of virus in saliva is thought to be so small that the risk is extremely low.
- Sharing your fantasies with each other. 'Talking dirty' can be great fun and on its own obviously carries no risks!

How to look after yourself

The most important point is to be aware of the risks you might be running. At least you then have the option to protect yourself and, if you think you've had risky sex, to get medical advice.

Partners

The more partners you have, the more risks you could be running. Unsafe sex between men and women was defined in one study as having two or more partners in the last year and never using a condom during that time.

In the Durex Report 2001, people were asked whether the risk of HIV had changed their behaviour. For some it had; 21 per cent now had only one sexual partner and 17 per cent were more careful about their choice of partner. Fewer partners and being careful about who you sleep with reduces risk.

Some people think that it's only people who sleep around who are at risk and that there's no need to use condoms if you have a series of steady relationships. This isn't true.

It's possible to get an infection even if you're in a stable, long-term relationship and both of you are faithful to each other. Of course the risks are minimal, though not non-existent, because one of you could have had an infection for a long time without being aware of it. You could also get genital herpes after having oral sex if your partner has a cold sore.

23

Partner checks

Before you start having sex

Before becoming close sexually, it's a good idea to try to find out more about your partner's sexual past; for instance, how many partners they've had, and whether they've ever had an STI. Obviously you're treading on delicate ground here. You need to be sensitive about how you do this, and to know how and when to bring up the subject in a non-threatening way so that your partner doesn't feel insulted by your questions. Clearly this isn't always easy and the second part of this chapter suggests ways of going about this and discusses the issues in more detail.

- If you suspect your partner has had unprotected sex with other people, visits prostitutes or is a drug user and shares needles, then your potential risk of contracting a STI is high.
- If you're about to have sex and notice that your partner has signs of infection (e.g. rashes, sores or discharge) then don't go any further, explain your concerns and say you think it's a good idea for your partner to go to a sexual health clinic to get checked out.
- Some partners decide to visit a clinic together before becoming sexually intimate with each other in order to get the all clear, and see this as a mark of respect for each other.

Genital health

It's easier to get an infection if genital skin is damaged or broken, so aim to keep your skin clean and healthy. Avoid scented products, which may irritate the skin. Women shouldn't douche (wash out the vagina), as this can cause various vaginal problems by upsetting the pH (chemical) balance and mix of healthy bacteria in the vagina. Similarly men shouldn't wash with any products that irritate their genitals.

If you're thinking about body-piercing in the genital area get it done properly, with safe sterile equipment, follow aftercare instructions to keep the pierced area clean and dry, and get medical advice if the skin becomes infected.

Before penetrative sex make sure you're well lubricated and avoid any lubricants or products that irritate and damage your skin.

Barrier protection

At the moment the most important safeguard is using condoms.

Condoms

Male and female condoms not only act as contraceptives, but also provide good protection against HIV and other STIs, although they're less able to protect against skin-to-skin infections such as genital warts and herpes because condoms don't cover all potentially infected skin.

Condoms need to be used correctly and every time you have sex. If they break, slip, fall off or aren't put on correctly you won't be protected, so contact a sexual health clinic for advice.

In the Durex Report 2001, 13 per cent of people said they didn't like using condoms and 7 per cent said partners didn't like them. If you think that condoms are boring and a killjoy, think again. They're getting sexier, available in all sorts of sizes, colours and flavours as well as thicknesses. Most condoms are made of rubber; plastic ones (Avanti) are thinner and odourless, described as feeling more natural and may be the answer if you or your partner feel that condoms reduce sensation.

There are lots of types of condoms, which means you should be able to find a product that suits you and your partner. They're widely available from all sorts of shops and places including pharmacies and supermarkets, and you may be able to get them free from family planning and sexual health clinics, and also from Brook Advisory Centres. (You can get various products by mail order and I've included details of 'Sexware' in Chapter 8.)

Contraceptives, such as the female cap or diaphragm, which are placed over the neck of the womb (the cervix), to stop sperm entering the womb, offer some but less protection against STIs so aren't a substitute for a condom.

What do people know about condoms and infection protection?

Key findings from the Durex Report 2001 include:

- Most people (nine out of ten) know condoms can help to protect against HIV infection;

- But only 28 per cent know that condoms help protect against chlamydia, one of the commonest STIs;
- However, six out of ten know condoms can protect against syphilis and gonorrhoea;
- 16- to 24-year-olds were less aware of how condoms can protect against a range of STIs, and men were also generally less aware than women.

The male condom

- *Lubricants* – most condoms are already lubricated, which helps to stop the condom tearing, but use more if you feel uncomfortable. Don't use oil-based lubricants such as baby oil, or Vaseline or massage oils on rubber condoms as this can damage them. Instead use water-based lubricants like KY Jelly – ask the pharmacist for details of the range of water-based ones. Sylk – a new lubricant derived from the kiwi fruit – is gentle, non-irritating and odourless and can be used with all condoms. It's available from Sexware (see Chapter 8) or ring 01923 285544 or see www.sylk.co.uk for details.
- *Anal sex* – use a stronger condom (e.g. Durex Ultra Strong) and plenty of lubricant to stop the condom tearing. Change the condom if you're going to then have vaginal sex to stop bacteria from the anus getting into the vagina.
- *Rubber allergy* – condoms can cause problems if you're allergic to rubber. Make sure you're using a low-allergy rubber condom or switch to a plastic condom (e.g. Avanti), which is made of very thin plastic but may be a bit more expensive than a rubber one. You can use any sort of lubricant with plastic condoms.
- *Spermicides* – such as nonoxynol-9 – used with a condom can increase protection against infections, and some condoms also have a spermicidal lubricant added to them. But allergy to spermicides is quite common and can cause damage and inflammation in the genital tissues, which could actually make it easier for an STI to be transmitted. If you're allergic it's best not to use a spermicide unless you can find one that doesn't cause inflammation, and to use condoms that have a non-spermicidal

lubricant (see the Sexware catalogue). For more information about this ask for advice from a sexual health clinic.

- *Good quality condoms* – in the UK every pack of condoms must have the European CE mark but also look out for the British Standards kitemark BS EN 600. Don't use a condom if it's past its expiry date.
- *Storage* – keep condoms in a dry cool place as heat can damage them.
- *Use* – always use a new one every time.

How to use a condom

Practise!

Condoms should be easy and comfortable to use but it's tricky when you start using a condom, and lots of people end up having unprotected sex because they don't like them or find them difficult to put on.

In Zoe Seymour's article about having sex for the first time, 'Sex in the 21st Century' (*Independent*, 6 March 2001), Neil aged 17 explained that he abandoned condoms the first time he had sex. 'They were just too much of a turn-off. I knew how to use them thanks to my dad's embarrassing tuition but once we tried them it ruined the experience.'

Rick aged 19 made a similar point.

Nobody tells you condoms are difficult to use, that they can totally kill your erection. The first time I had sex it really worried me. I thought I was doing something wrong or was impotent. They should explain in sex education that you have to persevere with condoms.

The answer is not to put condoms to one side but to recognize that most people find it difficult to put condoms on to start with.

Practice makes perfect. Practise using condoms until you feel really comfortable and confident about using them – that is, it's second nature to put one on. Men can practise using one when they masturbate. Putting on a condom can also seem off-putting and rather mechanical if you or your partner leaves the room to do this, so explore how to make condom-use part of a sexy, sensual experience. Women can learn how to put a condom on their male partner by practising on a banana or a cucumber or a sex toy.

Follow instructions on the packet carefully. Here's how to avoid common mistakes.

Before penetration
- Remove the condom carefully from the packet – condoms can be torn accidentally by sharp fingernails or jewellery.
- Put the condom on when the penis is hard and before there is any contact between the penis and your partner's body because fluid release early on from the penis can contain not only lots of sperm but also STIs.
- Make sure the condom is the right way round and not inside out; the rolls should be on the outside and not the inside of the condom.
- Putting it on – with one hand place the condom on the top of the penis by squeezing the closed end of the condom between finger and thumb to make sure there's no air in the condom.
- Unroll the condom all the way down to the bottom of the penis.

Afterwards
- After you've ejaculated (come off) withdraw the penis when it's still hard, holding the condom at the base of the penis to make sure it stays on. Remove the condom only when the penis is fully withdrawn, keep the penis and condom away from your partner.
- Get rid of the condom by wrapping it in tissue and throwing it away. Don't flush it down the toilet. Never use a condom more than once.

The female condom

For details of Femidom – the female condom – see the website: www.female.condom.org

Some women prefer to use this because it makes them feel more in control but some men dislike it; others have complained that it's like a plastic bag; and some couples think it's noisy. Even though it's not to everyone's liking it's definitely worth checking it out to see what you and your partner feel about it, though it's more expensive than the male condom. You need to learn how to insert it properly but again practice makes perfect.

Its advantages include the fact that because it covers a bit more of the external genitals it may give you more protection against skin-to-skin infections such as herpes and genital warts, and it also protects the vagina against damage; it doesn't need extra lubrication and your partner doesn't have to withdraw straight after ejaculation as with the male condom. Also, you shouldn't have an allergic reaction to it since it's made of plastic not rubber.

But you need to be careful that the penis goes inside the condom and not down the side of it – guide your partner's penis during entry into the vagina to make sure it goes inside the condom – and you need to learn how to remove the condom correctly to make sure that semen doesn't spill onto your genitals.

Here's what the manufacturer's booklet says about the female condom:

- It's a strong, loose-fitting polyurethane (a soft, thin, odourless plastic) sheath about 6.5 inches long with a flexible ring at each end. It's inserted before sex into the vagina. The inner ring is used to insert the condom and help keep it in place; the outer ring is soft and stays on the outside of the vagina during sex.
- Since it's not rubber it doesn't cause allergic reactions.
- It's pre-lubricated with a non-spermicidal silicone-based lubricant to ease insertion and to make sex smoother.
- You don't need to take it out immediately after your partner has ejaculated.

Be prepared

Always carry condoms with you. This is sensible, good practice and doesn't mean you're promiscuous; rather that you're being responsible. In the Durex survey 17 per cent of people had unprotected sex because condoms weren't available.

Spermicides

The main protection against STIs comes from the male or female condom. I've mentioned before that using additional spermicide can increase protection but only if you're not allergic to it. If you're allergic, a spermicide may cause irritation to the vagina or penis and could do more harm than good by damaging the skin, making it easier for an infection to be transmitted. Double-check with a sexual health clinic but the usual advice if you're allergic is not to use additional spermicide.

Oral sex

Lots of couples enjoy oral sex, when the mouth and tongue are used to stimulate the genitals, but there is some degree of risk. Catching infections such as chlamydia and gonorrhoea through oral sex with an infected partner is possible, as is getting HIV though there is a smaller level of risk.

Oral sex is much less risky than unprotected penetrative sex but to reduce your risk further it is wise to use barrier protection. For oral sex on the penis, use a condom (spermicide can taste unpleasant so use an unlubricated condom or one that isn't lubricated with a spermicide). For oral sex with a woman place a 'dental dam' – a piece of rubber that's about 6 inches square – over her genitals. Dental dams are so-called because dentists use them to protect their faces from secretions from patients' mouths. You can buy dental dams or cut a condom into a square – experiment.

- Keep your mouth in good condition and get gum disease treated. Any cuts, bleeding gums, sores or other infections in your mouth, or recent dental surgery can make transmission of HIV more likely. Don't floss your teeth just before or after oral sex in case you cut the gums, and don't use a mouthwash during this time as it removes substances in saliva that may protect against HIV transmission.
- If you have unprotected oral sex, not 'coming off' in your partner's mouth may lessen the risk of HIV transmission, though fluid released before ejaculation can still transmit the virus.

Anal sex

Use stronger condoms and plenty of lubrication for penetrative anal sex (i.e. when the penis enters the anus).

Oral-anal sex – licking round the anus with your mouth and tongue, known as 'rimming' – is common among gay men, but some heterosexual couples also enjoy this. Again some STIs such as

30

hepatitis A may be passed on through this activity, so make sure the anus is clean, and for extra protection use a dental dam – apart from hepatitis A you could get infected by other organisms in the gut.

If you insert fingers into your partner's anus be careful because the inside of the anus is very delicate and can be damaged by sharp nails. There's a very small risk that infections such as hepatitis B could be transmitted if, for instance, you have a cut on your hand (normally the skin there provides a very good barrier against infection) and anal tissue is bleeding. To play safe use latex (rubber surgical-style) gloves and wash your hands afterwards. (Latex gloves are available from Sexware; see p. 99 for details.)

Hands

Remember that hands can spread certain infections, though the risk of this is low. If you want all the protection you can get, use rubber gloves if you're touching your partner's genital and anal area and wash your hands afterwards.

Sex toys

As mentioned earlier if you share sex toys make sure the toy is cleaned and covered in a new condom between use.

Alcohol and drugs

Watch out as too much alcohol and binge-drinking or taking recreational drugs may mean you end up doing something you regret later (e.g. having unprotected sex). In the Durex Report 2001, 23 per cent of people failed to use a condom because they got carried away and 15 per cent said they were too drunk to think about it. Drugs and alcohol can make you irresponsible, make it hard to think properly and mean you throw caution to the winds.

Holidays

- Going away on holiday to a foreign place where the sun shines all the time, where you relax and feel carefree may mean you end up doing things you would never dream of doing at home, such as having unprotected sex.

- Safer sex is particularly important when you're abroad. HIV exists all over the world but far more people are HIV infected in countries such as Spain and Italy than the UK, and in African countries such as Kenya about one in four adults has HIV.
- Make sure you're protected and take condoms with you. If you don't, you may find you can't get one when you need it and you may also find that you can't get the same quality condoms you're used to here. If you use the female condom, take this with you as you may not be able to get it in other countries.
- Insist on condom protection. If someone says that it's against their culture to use a condom, stick to your guns and explain that it's against your culture not to use one.

Vaccinations

In the future vaccinations may well play an important part in providing protection against STIs. Research trials are looking at how effective vaccinations are, for instance against the various human papilloma viruses, some of which cause genital warts.

Meanwhile there are vaccinations for hepatitis A and B. (See the sections on those infections in Chapter 6.) Hepatitis B is much more infectious than HIV and the Department of Health's new National Strategy on Sexual Health document says that more people are to be offered the hepatitis B vaccine in sexual health clinics.

Cervical smears

Cervical smears are offered to women aged 20 to 64 at three- to five-yearly intervals and play an important part in sexual health. There is a well-established link between the human papilloma virus (HPV) and cervical cancer. HPV causes genital warts although the types of HPV responsible for genital warts aren't normally responsible for cervical cancer (see the section on genital warts, pp. 51–6). There's now a trial scheme going on to test abnormal smear results for HPV infection and if the test is positive you'll be referred straightaway for further treatment.

The IUD

I discussed this in Chapter 2 (see p. 76). It's not a good idea having one fitted if your sexual lifestyle makes you more at risk of getting infections travelling up into the pelvic cavity.

When can you stop using protection?

Safer sex is all about reducing your risks with a new partner but lots of couples in long-term relationships don't use it. So when can you forget about safer sex? When you're absolutely sure you and your partner aren't infected, neither of you is having unprotected sex with someone else and neither of you shares drug-injecting equipment with anyone. But since it can be difficult to know you're in the 'all clear', some couples decide to get checked out at a sexual health clinic and take this as a mark of their commitment to each other.

Getting pregnant

Some STIs can cause problems in pregnancy and affect the health of your baby so unless you're both sure you're uninfected, it's a good idea for both of you to go to a clinic to get the 'all clear' before you stop using protection.

Screening

As from 2002 there will be a national screening programme for chlamydia for certain groups of young women (see the section on chlamydia on pp. 44–51). In 1999 the Department of Health introduced a policy to offer and recommend HIV testing to all pregnant women. In the National Strategy for Sexual Health document, routine HIV testing is to be offered in all sexual health clinics (see the section on HIV on pp. 75–80).

What if you're lesbian, gay or bisexual?

Lesbians

- There seems to be less research into the risks of STIs for lesbians but sex between women is generally thought to be comparatively less risky, and low risk for HIV because of low concentrations of the virus in vaginal secretions, though menstrual blood is more infectious.

- But infections such as herpes and genital warts can be passed on through skin-to-skin contact and, for some unknown reason bacterial vaginosis is quite common in lesbians. If you've had unprotected sex with men in the past you could also have one or more infections from that contact.

- So safer sex practices are still important. Use dental dams for oral sex and make sure that sex toys are covered with a new condom before they're used by each partner. If you have sex with a man, use protection.

- Some clinics run sessions for lesbians, so ask what's available and if there are information leaflets for lesbians.

Gay and bisexual men

- Sex between men remains the main route for HIV being passed on within the UK, according to the Public Health Laboratory Service.

- The latest figures show that for gay and bisexual men cases of gonorrhoea rose by 45 per cent between 1999 and 2000. There were 300 cases of syphilis in 2000, which is a tiny figure but it's alarming because it's an increase of 55 per cent since 1999. The cases have been among gay men mainly, and oral sex played an important part in spreading the disease.

- A 1999 study of gay men found that over half of those under 20 didn't use a condom.

- Diagnostic tests for men who have sex with men will also include a throat swab for gonorrhoea, a sample taken from the rectum if you're the one penetrated during anal sex, and screening for hepatitis B if you're not vaccinated against it.

- Safer sex means using condoms to protect yourself from HIV and other STIs, such as hepatitis B. Use plenty of water-based lubricants and stronger condoms for anal sex to reduce the risk of the condom breaking.

- Use latex gloves for 'fisting' (putting your hand in your partner's anus) as a general protection method for both of you. As I said in the section on anal sex, the lining of the anus is very delicate and can be cut easily by sharp nails, so, first, a glove reduces damage

34

to the lining and, second, reduces the small risk of an infection being passed either way; for instance, if you've also got a cut on your hand.

- Use condoms for oral sex – figures now indicate that between 3 and 8 per cent of cases of HIV among gay men are contracted through oral sex.
- Use dental dams for 'rimming' and be aware that apart from picking up an infection like hepatitis A from contact with faeces you may also pick up organisms from the gut.
- Keep sex toys clean and put a new condom on before sharing them.
- Ask at your local sexual health clinic about vaccinations for hepatitis A and B.
- Read *The Manual*, a gay men's guide to STIs; and *Safer Sex*, both available from the Terrence Higgins Trust (see Chapter 8).

What safer sex isn't

- The contraceptive pill – the pill doesn't protect against STIs.
- Withdrawing just before 'coming off', pre-ejaculate fluid can contain infectious organisms.
- Urinating and washing after sex.

The things that stop safer sex

One of the reasons people often don't practise safer sex is simply because they don't know how to talk about it or are too embarrassed to bring up the subject. Yes, you can use a condom without talking about the issues behind condom use but safer sex also means knowing more about your partner's attitudes to sex, their sexual history and sexual practices; all of which means talking about sex.

It takes confidence to do this. For many people it's even more difficult to talk about these things if they've just become sexually active because they're caught up with so many other things that they're trying to understand and deal with.

So what gets in the way of safer sex? Certain ideas, thoughts and feelings about what sex is all about play a big part here, and what I've done in the rest of this chapter is to bring these out into the open so that you can see what they are and make up your mind.

Sex should be passionate and spontaneous

The idea that sex should be passionate and spontaneous is a very powerful one. Sex – making love – should be wild, exciting, out of control, urgent, overwhelming and irresistible if it's any good. Very often this is how it's shown in films and advertisements and written about in books.

So where does this leave safer sex, which involves a bit of planning and forethought? In the Durex Report 2001, 23 per cent of people surveyed said they had unprotected sex because they were 'caught up in the moment of passion'. Is it possible to have passionate sex if you practise safer sex?

The answer to this is a very definite 'yes', but it's something you need to have thought about, talked about and to be prepared for so that the practical aspects of safer sex can become part and parcel of your lovemaking and not things that disrupt sex.

Sharing safer-sex issues with your partner can mean you're much closer emotionally, which also makes for better sex. Also, you're likely to be more relaxed and not worrying about the consequences of risky sex, which again makes for better sex.

Take your time

One of the reasons that safer sex may not happen when you start a relationship is because there isn't time to discuss things, because you rush into sex.

Of course it's not true that people always leap into bed with each other straightaway, at the first opportunity. Studies on sexuality indicate that most people go through various stages of intimacy which can take weeks or months before they start having penetrative sex, according to Julia Cole in her book, *Find the Love of Your Life*.

The stages are kissing and cuddling, touching but not on the breast and genitals, followed by more intense kissing, then going on to total body contact, then intimate touching of the breasts and genitals, possibly mutual masturbation and finally sexual intercourse.

These stages give you time to get to know each other and to decide how far you want to go and whether you want to become sexually intimate, and the more you know each other the easier it's likely to be to talk about safer sex.

It's wrong-headed to think that passion and speed of intimacy automatically go together. The truth is that you're likely to have more satisfying sex with someone you can talk to openly about your fears, worries, sexual needs and dislikes and this usually takes time to happen. Sex can be incredibly satisfying when you know each other better and trust each other.

By taking your time and making this one of your golden rules, you'll have more opportunity to explore safer-sex issues when the time feels right instead of suddenly having to rush into the subject.

Talking about safer-sex issues before you become sexually intimate will protect you, and you may decide as you find out more about the other person that for a whole load of reasons you don't want to have sex with them, after all. That's fine.

Rushing into sex doesn't mean better sex. On the contrary, you may end up regretting it and worrying about the consequences, not least of which are the infection risks.

One-night stands

Partying and clubbing are high risk times for one-night stands. Alcohol fuels that sense that 'nothing matters', 'you can get away with anything' and 'wanting to lose control is OK'. It's best not to binge on alcohol for all sorts of reasons, not least because if both of you are drunk then sex won't be so good. But many of us do get drunk at some time or other. Be prepared: always have condoms with you and make it your golden rule that you'll use them, no matter what.

It should feel like an automatic response to do this. Raise the issue with your partner while you've still got some clothes on. Explain that you never have sex without a condom and ask whether they want to use one of your condoms. Steer clear of them if they won't use a condom.

If you don't have condoms, the options are of course no sex, or the lower-risk sexual activities mentioned in the first part of this chapter, such as mutual masturbation or oral sex.

Thinking you're not at risk

It's easy to kid yourself that it's only other people who get infections so you don't need to use safer sex but, as I keep saying, this just isn't the case and anyone who's sexually active could get infected.

Feeling you have to have sex

When you start to become sexually active, you may feel intense pressures to have sex, from yourself – wanting to try this experience on which so much emphasis is placed – or feeling pressured to 'jump into bed' by your friends and feeling 'left out' if you don't. In this situation it's very easy to be confused about what you really want and for safer-sex issues to fly out of the window.

These pressures are very real, but rushing into sex too soon can lead to later regrets as well as worries. If you don't want sex then don't have it, and give yourself a pat on the back. In one survey of 16- to 24-year-olds, 15 per cent of men and 36 per cent of women felt they'd had sexual intercourse too soon, and the younger the age they'd first had sex the more likely they were to regret this.

It's important to recognize the power of other pressures. We live in a world where sex is used everywhere to sell all sorts of products. Once you realize what's happening and acknowledge this, these pressures won't seem so powerful and you'll be able to see them more for what they are, and make up your own mind about what you want to do.

Respect

Respect is vital to any relationship and means better sex. If someone puts pressure on you to have sex against your wishes, they don't respect you. If you lose this person because you weren't certain whether you wanted to have sex although they insisted, then it's for the best that you split up.

Low self-esteem

Feeling bad about yourself can also be another reason for ending up having sex. Underlying this is the thought that you're not worth anything, which can mean you find it hard to look after yourself, which in turn means you don't practise safer sex.

You may feel grateful that someone is showing an interest in you, however suspect that interest is. Beware of anyone who says things like, 'If you loved me you'd have sex with me' or 'You're frigid'. Challenge these ideas and ask yourself what sort of person would say that to get you into bed. The answer is someone who doesn't have your best interests at heart. If you don't want sex then don't have it. Consider whether you want to go on with this relationship and to have your confidence undermined in this way. You might find it helpful to see a counsellor to talk about how you feel about yourself and how you can stand up for yourself.

Trust

You may think that you can't talk about safer sex because your partner will think you don't trust them, even though you know that it's the right thing to do. In fact asking these questions implies that you do respect and trust your partner to take your concerns seriously. Explain that you're not implying that they sleep around; the fact of the matter is that being sexually active carries risks with it. If your partner cares about you they'll appreciate you've brought up the subject and probably be relieved that you've raised a subject of concern to you both.

Talking about safer sex

Communication is hard for most of us, and sexual communication is even harder. Some people may find sex easy to talk about but most of us don't, for all sorts of reasons. Sex can still be an embarrassing subject: talking about intimate parts of the body isn't something that many of us find easy and then there are all the feelings that go with it.

For many people, talking about sex feels like walking across a minefield that could explode at any moment if you put a foot in the wrong place. All of which means that many of us find, particularly when we're new to sex, that we just don't know how to talk about sex, let alone safer-sex issues.

What words do you use and when and how should you do this without insulting your partner? These are the sorts of thoughts that most of us have when we think about how to bring up the subject. Many people find this so off-putting that it's tempting to forget the whole business.

The truth is that it's not easy to start, and it takes time and practice to learn how to do this. But the more you do this the easier it becomes, and most partners will be grateful to you for bringing up the topic.

Some tips
- The best way to communicate about this is to choose the right moment, one when you both feel fresh and not stressed. If you take time to find out about each other you'll have opportunities when the time feels right. Bring up the subject when you're both relaxed and comfortable, have plenty of time and don't feel too pressured by other demands.
- Bring up the subject before you start having sex. It's pretty difficult to sort this out once you're in bed and physically and emotionally aroused. Talk about it over a coffee or a meal, somewhere private where you can go over the issues.
- Think about what you want to say beforehand (things to cover include: whether you could be putting your partner at risk for any STIs and vice versa; whether either of you has a chronic STI such as herpes; whether to get tested for infections before you start having sex; using condoms every time you have sex).
- If you're finding it difficult, say so – if you're honest and open about how you're feeling it'll help. Try to put yourself in your partner's shoes so that you can find the right words to use, which won't be antagonizing. Don't make blanket statements such as 'People who don't use safe sex are stupid'. Instead edge your way into the subject, go gently, explain your concerns and then ask your partner something like 'How do you feel about what I've said?' which allows them to respond.
- Aim to raise the subject in a way that comes over as helpful and non-critical. It's all too easy to rush into the subject, blurt out some things and leave your partner feeling confused and upset. Check that they've understood what you've said, as it's very easy for there to be misunderstandings and for your partner not to have heard properly what you're saying.

Hopefully you'll find your partner is glad you brought up the subject. But you could get an angry response not because they don't care about you but because they think you're criticizing them. If this happens try to explain again, perhaps using different words. Say that you're not having a go but need to talk about this to safeguard their health and your own.

Give your partner information and time to think things over. They might want some leaflets about STIs to look through. Some people may want to do this in their own time and space so that the information has time to sink in.

But if your partner is adamant that safer sex is rubbish, that there's no need for it, or that it's unmanly or against their religion, think carefully about whether you really want to have sex with someone who could be putting not only your short-term but also your long-term health at risk.

Talking about condoms

Most people find condoms awkward to use, as we discussed in the first part of this chapter. Learn to talk about condoms, the ones you like and how to make them sexy and not a turn-off. Putting one on can seem very mechanical if you or your partner leaves the room to do this: instead experiment and explore ways of putting on a condom that are sensual and sexual.

How to argue for safer sex

In her excellent book *Sexually Transmitted Diseases*, Lisa Marr talks about the sorts of things that people sometimes say when they argue that safer sex isn't necessary. She suggests ways of challenging these thoughts:

- 'You don't need safe sex if you're in love'. Answer – being in love won't protect you against STIs.
- 'Condoms spoil the pleasure'. Answer – find condoms that suit you, there are lots of options. Also not using a condom spoils pleasure because you're worrying about the consequences of unprotected sex.
- 'Talking about safer sex means you've slept around'. Answer – no, it doesn't. It means you want to protect your and your partner's health and that you're well informed. People who don't talk about safer sex just don't know what the real facts are.
- 'A condom isn't necessary if the man withdraws before he comes off'. Answer – no, this isn't true, because before a man comes off

he releases small amounts of pre-ejaculate, which can pass on infection.

- 'Sex is better and more spontaneous when a condom isn't used'. Answer – not true because sex is better when we're both relaxed and it won't be if one or both of us is worrying about the consequences of unprotected sex.
- 'I don't use condoms and I don't have STIs because I don't have any symptoms'. Answer – the fact you don't have symptoms doesn't mean you're free of infections.
- 'Show me you really care about me by not using a condom'. Answer – I do care about you and that means using condoms to protect my health and yours.

Talking to your partner about a chronic infection

Some infections, such as genital warts and herpes, are chronic and may flare up from time to time. They can't be cured as such, so how do you discuss this with a potential new partner if you have one of these infections?

It's not easy but it's best to do this before you become sexually intimate. Give your partner as much information as possible about the STI, the chances of passing it on, and what can be done to try and reduce transmission risks (e.g. not having sex at those times when herpes is active).

Being honest and open usually brings partners together rather than pulling them apart and your partner is likely to appreciate your honesty; whereas they may feel betrayed, angry and hurt if you mention it later on once you've started having sex.

If you want help about how to bring up the issues and the words to use, you may find that you can talk things through with a health adviser at a sexual health clinic. It sometimes helps to do a role play with the adviser playing the part of your partner so you can practise how to raise and talk about the subject, and also to reverse roles to see how it feels from your partner's viewpoint.

Once you've raised the subject your partner may well want time to think things through, want as much information as possible about the STI and may want to see a health adviser as well for more information. Give your partner time to do these things and don't think you're being rejected.

But prepare yourself in advance for the possibility that your partner may not want to continue the relationship.

Finally

Julia Cole explores all sorts of issues to do with relationships including safer sex in her book, *Find the Love of Your Life*. I've ended this chapter with some important points she makes:

- Safer sex is not only about taking precautions, 'It's also a by-product of thinking through your personal approach to sex and how you feel about beginning your sex life with a new partner.'
- Feel ready – don't start having sex just to please your partner or because you feel under pressure.
- Take your time – 'Most people who race into sexual relationships regret taking this action.' Drugs and alcohol often fuel the rush into sex, and someone who seemed very attractive in the night may look a lot less desirable in the morning.
- Be intuitive – listen to your gut feeling about whether someone is trustworthy or not to be trusted.

4

Common Sexually Transmitted Infections

This chapter looks at four of the commonest STIs in alphabetical order: chlamydia, genital warts, gonorrhoea and herpes, and expands on material covered in earlier chapters.

Chlamydia

What is it?

Chlamydia is an infection caused by a bacterium – *Chlamydia trachomatis* – which is passed on through sexual contact (i.e. by unprotected vaginal, anal or oral sex), and which usually affects the genitals (most commonly the cervix in women and the urethra in both men and women), though it can also affect the throat and rectum and it can be spread by the fingers from the genitals to the eyes. It's estimated that there's a 66 per cent chance of the infection being passed on between regular sexual partners. Chlamydia can also be passed from a mother to her baby at birth.

People who have chlamydia often have other STIs, in particular gonorrhoea. It's now clear that chlamydia is very often responsible for non-specific urethritis (NSU) where the urethra (the tube through which urine is excreted) becomes inflamed.

How common is it?

Chlamydia is one of the commonest infections and the number of cases continues to climb. In 1999, 56,855 people were diagnosed with what is called 'straightforward chlamydial infection'; in other words, it hasn't caused complications, such as moving upwards into the womb and other pelvic organs. Figures have increased to 62,565 in 2000, an increase of 19 per cent for men and 17 per cent for women.

Who gets it?

Anyone can get chlamydia, including older people. For instance, figures for 1999 show that 39 men and 9 women in the over-64 age group were diagnosed as having a chlamydial infection.

But you're much more likely to get it if you're young and especially if you're under 24, sexually active and don't use condoms or if you've recently changed sexual partners – at least one in 14 young people has chlamydia. The increase in figures is probably not just to do with people having unprotected sex but because there's better awareness of the disease and detection tests are improving.

Are there any symptoms?

One of the most important points about chlamydia is that often there aren't any symptoms; 70 per cent of cases are symptomless. Only a minority of people develop symptoms. Women in particular often don't get any warnings, and it's become increasingly clear as more is discovered about this disease (which people became more aware of in the early 1970s) that men are often symptomless, too.

Symptoms can appear from one to three weeks after exposure to the infection but may not appear for months, years or possibly a lifetime, or may be so mild as to be unnoticed. If your partner develops symptoms you may feel very confused and upset and think they've been unfaithful to you, but the infection could be a legacy from a previous relationship.

Symptoms of uncomplicated infections

Uncomplicated infections are those where the infection hasn't developed into something more serious.

Both sexes

An infection in the rectum rarely has symptoms but there may be a discharge and some discomfort. Throat infections (which usually occur from performing oral sex on an infected man) rarely produce symptoms and if they do may manifest as a bit of throat irritation. Red, sore, itchy eyes will occur if you get conjunctivitis, which is an eye infection.

Women

You probably won't have any (about 80 per cent of women are symptomless). When they occur symptoms include vaginal discharge, an inflamed cervix, bleeding in between periods or after sex, lower abdominal pain, a swollen, sore rectum, pain when you pee (don't assume this is cystitis or due to bruising of the urethra during sex or to an infection with *E. coli* bacteria from the bowel, as chlamydia can irritate the urethra).

Men

It's becoming increasingly clear that many men – as many as one in two – have no symptoms; if you do, your symptoms are likely to include pain when urinating and a discharge from the tip of the penis.

Uncomplicated cases of chlamydia can normally be successfully treated and cured with antibiotics, but people often don't get treated because they don't realize they have an infection, and this means that complications and long-term problems are very likely to occur.

Cases of complicated chlamydial infection

Women

Women are particularly affected by this in a number of ways. If the infection moves further up into the pelvis it can result in pelvic inflammatory disease (PID) which, depending on its severity, may cause a lot of pain and discomfort as well as infertility – you may not find it easy to get pregnant. Around one in three women with an untreated infection develops PID.

The cervix (neck of the womb), womb and Fallopian tubes can get infected, which can result in blocked Fallopian tubes, causing infertility. If your tubes are affected and you get pregnant there's a greater chance that the embryo develops in the tube in what's known as an 'ectopic' ('out of place') pregnancy because a pregnancy should develop in the womb. Ectopic pregnancies are not only painful but also life-threatening because the tube may burst, causing serious bleeding. It's thought that as many as 40 per cent of ectopic pregnancies are caused by chlamydia.

If you become pregnant you may miscarry because of the infection, or it can be passed to your baby at birth. About 60 per cent of babies born to mothers with chlamydia get infected, with about a third of babies developing conjunctivitis (sticky red eyes). About a fifth of infected babies will develop pneumonia, usually between four and 12 weeks after birth.

Men

For men, the commonest complication of chlamydia is epididymitis (a red, swollen testicle is a sign of this), which is a painful infection of the epididymis – the tube which carries sperm from the testicle. If untreated, epididymitis may reduce fertility by stopping the movement of sperm, because inflammation can cause scarring by blocking the sperm transport system.

A less common complication, which affects men more than women, is called 'Reiter's syndrome'. Symptoms include: urethral problems, joint inflammation, conjunctivitis and skin rashes.

Can chlamydia cause cervical cancer?

At the start of 2001 there was a research report in the *Journal of the American Medical Association* (January 2001, vol. 285, no. 1), of a study where blood samples had been taken from 530,000 Scandinavian women. The results found that several strains of chlamydia, in particular type G, seemed to be linked to the later development of cervical cancer.

These results don't mean that it's been proved that the G strain of chlamydia *causes* cervical cancer; only that there may be some sort of link, though the exact nature of this link has yet to be established. More research is needed into this; meanwhile it's important not to ignore possible warning signs of cervical problems, such as bleeding after sex and bleeding in between periods. Get checked out if you're worried, have your regular smear checks and use safer-sex measures all the time.

Testing for chlamydia

It should be possible to detect the infection about seven to 14 days after exposure to it, so if you're tested too early the infection may not show up. Get advice from the clinic on this – if you think you may only just have been exposed to it, the clinic will advise on the right time to do the tests.

There have been lots of problems in the past about the best way to detect this infection, and concern that tests weren't showing it up, but the outlook is improving. For both men and women there seems to be a good, simple test using urine samples, which seems to be highly accurate, although no test is 100 per cent accurate.

47

For best results, you shouldn't urinate for two hours before having the test to make sure enough organisms are in the urine – get advice from the clinic about this before you turn up there. Swabs may also be taken from the cervix and urethra in women or from the urethra in men. Swabs may also be taken from the throat and anus. The time it takes to get results will vary depending on the tests done but is often about a week.

Can you be screened for chlamydia?

Since chlamydia can cause such damage and because it's so often symptomless, you may wonder whether you can be screened for it at regular intervals as a preventive measure, in the same way that women have regular cervical smears. At the time of writing there isn't any routine screening for this infection but that looks set to change in the not-too-distant future.

In Scandinavia screening for this infection is thought to have significantly reduced the risk of infertility and ectopic pregnancy. As a result, in 1999 the Department of Health in the UK set up a pilot project in one part of the country to screen women aged 16 to 24 for the infection. They were offered a simple urine test to check for the infection if they were visiting their GP for some reason or other (not necessarily anything to do with an STI).

The results have been analysed to see if it makes sense to have a nationwide screening programme. Early results show that about one in 10 of those tested had this silent infection.

The Department of Health announced in its National Strategy for Sexual Health document that a programme of screening for chlamydia would begin for at-risk groups in 2002. In the document the Department of Health says that about 10 per cent of sexually active young women are likely to be infected. The screening programme will be offered initially to certain groups of young women: for example, those having their first cervical smear, or those women requesting an abortion or attending a sexual health clinic). The screening programme will be widened later on to include other groups.

There was also a news report in 2001 that a company was developing a self-test kit for chlamydia for men.

How is chlamydia treated?

The treatment of uncomplicated cases of chlamydia is with antibiotics. Treatment with antibiotics is highly successful but needs to be done as soon as possible to stop the risk of permanent damage that can occur if the infection remains untreated.

There's a choice of antibiotics. One of the best is doxycycline, of which the recommended dosage is usually 100mg twice a day for seven days; or you may be prescribed a single 1g dose of another drug, azithromycin. If these medicines don't work you may be given others (e.g. ofloxacin taken once or twice a day usually for seven days). The choice of drug treatment also depends on whether you have another STI, such as gonorrhoea.

Ask what the treatment options are, how often drugs have to be taken, how long for, what side-effects to expect and whether you can do anything to lessen side-effects. For instance, some drugs can cause stomach upset so you may be advised to take the medicine at meal times to lessen the risk. Some may cause dental staining; some may make you more sensitive to sunlight, in which case you need to ask how to cope with this. Check whether your drug interacts in any way with other medicines or products you're taking, as some drugs may not be so well absorbed if taken with milk or antacids.

Taking doxycycline may mean the combined contraceptive pill doesn't work so well for the time you're taking it and seven days afterwards. (See below – you shouldn't have sex during treatment but if you do this is another reason why you should use a condom: to protect you not only against reinfection and other STIs but to protect you against an unwanted pregnancy.)

If your throat is also infected you shouldn't need extra treatment but once treatment is finished a throat swab should be taken to make sure the infection has gone.

It's very important to see treatment through to the end and to take it exactly as instructed. Ask in advance what you should do if you develop side-effects (e.g. vomiting so that you can't keep the medicine down) or if you forget to take a dose. Double-check this, but with doxycycline the normal advice is that you should take the dose as soon as you remember but if you don't remember until you're about to take your next dose, just take the next dose as usual and don't double-up.

Complications

A combination of antibiotics is given for a longer time for problems like PID in women and epididymitis in men.

Pregnancy

If you're pregnant you can't take doxycycline. Alternatives may include erythromycin – usually 500mg four times a day for seven days – but this can have significant side-effects and many people get nausea and vomiting. Another option that your medical adviser might suggest is to have smaller amounts of the drug but for a longer period of time (e.g. 500mg twice a day for 14 days).

Retesting

Ask whether you need to be tested afterwards to see if you're cured. This isn't always necessary because drugs like doxycycline are highly effective, but you may need to be retested if there's any chance you could have been reinfected or if you still have symptoms. If you're pregnant you should be retested after treatment to make sure the infection is eliminated so it can't be passed on to your baby at birth.

Testing to see if you're clear of infection shouldn't be done for at least three weeks after you've finished treatment. Tests done too soon may give false-positive results because dead bacteria are still present and may show you as having an infection when you don't.

What about sex during treatment?

It's important not to have sex during treatment in case you get reinfected, even if using a condom because condoms can't guarantee 100 per cent protection. Ask when you can safely start to have sex again.

What about partners?

It's vital that you don't infect other people or get reinfected because your sexual partner has chlamydia. Your current partner and past ones over the last six months or possibly longer need to be told they might have an infection and that they need to get tested. Normal practice is to offer treatment regardless of test results because of the risk that they may test negative but still have an infection. A health adviser will work out with you who needs to be contacted and the best way to do this.

Genital warts

What are they and what causes them?

Warts are small outgrowths of skin caused by the human papilloma virus (HPV). There are over 90 types of the virus and around a third are acquired sexually. Warts can occur anywhere on the body but when they develop around the genitals – on or around the penis or vagina – they're called 'genital warts' and technically known as 'perianal warts' if they develop around the anus.

It's important to say that not much is understood about these warts, though more is being discovered as time goes by.

How common are they?

Genital warts were the most common STI diagnosed in sexual health clinics in 1999, when more than 70,000 men and women were diagnosed with genital warts for the first time. According to the latest figures for 2000, genital warts are still the commonest STI.

Who gets them?

Anyone can get them and it's estimated that over 50 per cent of sexually active adults have been infected, but according to the Public Health Laboratory Service those most likely to get these warts are women aged 16 to 24 and men aged 20 to 24. If you have unprotected sex, have more than one partner or change partners frequently then your risk of infection increases.

How do you get them?

Genital warts are spread through skin-to-skin contact and most easily transmitted to the thinner skin found on the vulva, vagina and cervix in women and on the penis and scrotum in men. Genital warts are passed on during vaginal or anal sex, though it's possible to get warts round the anus without having had anal sex.

About two-thirds of people who have sexual contact with someone who has these warts will develop them, generally within one to three months of contact. But obvious symptoms may not appear for several or many years, so if you've been with your partner for years and they develop warts it doesn't necessarily mean that they've been unfaithful to you as the infection could have been dormant for a long time.

You can develop warts in or around the mouth after oral sex if your partner has genital warts, although this is rare. It's also possible but very unlikely that the virus can be passed to the genitals from warts on fingers.

It's a small risk but if you're pregnant you can pass the virus to your baby at birth, which may occasionally result in the baby getting throat warts.

What are the symptoms?

- Fewer than 1 per cent of people develop obvious symptoms and you may not be aware that you've got any, but if you're symptomless you can still pass on the virus.
- When warts do appear they come in all sorts of sizes and shapes. They may be large or small, flat or raised, some coloured, hard or soft. They may be fleshy growths or pinkish-white, small lumps or larger cauliflower-shaped lumps, which you or your partner may notice. You may have one or several warts. The warts aren't painful though they can itch a bit, but you may be very upset by the appearance of the warts and want them removed for cosmetic reasons.
- Women can get warts on the inside and outside of the vagina and also on the cervix, which may cause slight bleeding or rarely an unusual, coloured, vaginal discharge. Men can get them on the tip or shaft of the penis or around the anus and occasionally on the scrotum.

How dangerous are warts? Can they cause cervical cancer?

There are mixed messages about this. Warts aren't dangerous and don't pose a threat to long-term health. On the other hand, it's now thought that 99 per cent of cervical cancers are linked in some way to the warts' virus (HPV), so how much should you worry about this if you have warts? The main point is that it's only certain strains of HPV that cause genital warts; most visible genital warts are caused by HPV types such as 6 and 11 but these aren't linked to cervical cancer.

The types linked to cervical cancer and other cancers in the genitals are known to be 16, 18 and 33. Other factors are also relevant; for example, if you smoke your risk of cervical cancer increases.

Genital warts aren't a big risk factor for developing cervical cancer but it's important to keep having your routine cervical smears. Current advice at the moment is that you don't need to have smears more often if you have warts.

If you have warts on the cervix it's normal for your doctor to do a colposcopy. This involves looking in more detail at the cervix with a special magnifying glass to see if there are any abnormal cell changes there. Sometimes a tissue sample known as a 'biopsy' will be taken so that cells can be looked at in more detail in the laboratory. (This doesn't happen automatically but research is being done at the moment to see whether women who have borderline smears – i.e. slightly abnormal ones – should be tested for HPV to see if they need to be sent straight away for a colposcopy rather than being monitored over a period of time.)

A vaccination against some of the HPV strains may be available in the not-too-distant future. A news report in the magazine *New Scientist* (3 March 2001) referred to a successful American trial using a vaccine based on HPV 16.

How are warts diagnosed?

Warts are diagnosed by looking at them. If they're not obvious, a weak vinegar-like solution is put on the outside of the genitals as this turns any warts white. The doctor may also check inside the vagina or anus to see if there are warts there. Further investigations will be needed if there are any concerns that the wart isn't a wart and is in fact some other sort of growth.

Since it's estimated that about 20 per cent of people with genital warts have other infections it's important to be screened for these too.

How are warts treated?

Genital warts are caused by a virus but you can't cure the virus itself and antibiotics won't have any effect. Treatments can get rid of the warts, though they may well return, and if your immune system isn't working well the warts may be more difficult to treat. The sort of treatment you have will depend on such factors as how many warts you have, the sorts of warts and where they are. Treatments all have side-effects so you need to ask about the pros and cons of each one and which one is best for you.

It's important to realize that warts don't need treatment unless they're irritating you or causing you discomfort. One of the main reasons warts are treated is for cosmetic reasons as some people are embarrassed by the warts because they think they're unsightly.

If you're not bothered by the warts, keep the genitals clean and dry and avoid using anything like perfumed soap and bubble baths, which might irritate them. Without treatment the warts may go away by themselves or they could stay the same or increase in size and number.

If you have treatment don't expect it to work first time round; recurrence rates are high particularly when the immune system isn't working so well, as I've said. The warts may also be more likely to return if you're stressed or smoke cigarettes. So don't be alarmed if you need several courses of treatment.

Treatments may cause discomfort but shouldn't be painful, and include podophyllin, which is painted onto the warts and washed off four hours later but it shouldn't be applied in excess or internally. Treatment takes place in the clinic once or twice weekly. Podophyllotoxin is a purified form of podophyllin that can be used at home. It's applied usually twice daily for three days followed by four days rest, for four cycles.

Trichloroacetic acid is normally applied weekly in the clinic but needs to be applied with care and the surrounding skin protected. The treatment may cause intense burning for about ten minutes after it's put on.

Another treatment is imiquimod (brand name Aldara) for external warts, a cream which works by triggering the immune system to react against the warts. Applied at night three times a week, it's washed off six to ten hours after application. A box normally contains 12 individual treatments. It usually takes two weeks before you notice any improvement and up to eight weeks for the warts to clear. Normally there's no point continuing with the treatment after eight weeks, though it can be used for up to 16 weeks. The cream shouldn't be used for internal warts or if there's a lot of pain and swelling around the warts, though it's normal to have some soreness when the cream is applied. Ask about when you can have sex if you are being treated with this drug. Usual advice is that you shouldn't use it if you're going to have sex within ten hours – the cream may damage rubber condoms and diaphragms.

Warts can also be destroyed by various methods such as by freezing or with a laser.

Warts won't be eradicated by antibiotics because they aren't caused by a bacterial infection. They should not be treated with self-help treatments designed for warts on the hands.

Pregnancy

It's important to tell the doctor if you're pregnant or trying to conceive because some of the treatments could harm the developing baby. Treatments like podophyllin or imiquimod aren't suitable but freezing treatments can be used. Another option may be to delay treatment until after the birth.

There's a very small risk of the virus being passed to the baby at birth so there's been a question about whether a Caesarean should be done, though current advice is that this isn't normally necessary.

What about sex during treatment?

Talk to the clinic about this. It'll depend obviously on how comfortable you feel and what sort of treatment you're having. Condoms offer some but not complete protection because they protect against the wart virus only if the affected area is covered, which it may not be, but remember that condoms still protect against other STIs. All in all it makes sense to use condoms, certainly during treatment and for several months afterwards.

Partners

The health adviser will discuss with you who should be contacted. Since your current sexual partner may have undetected warts and other infections, it may be a good idea for them to be checked out.

Gonorrhoea

What is it?

The 'clap', as gonorrhoea is commonly called, is a bacterial infection, *Neisseria gonorrhoeae*, which often affects the urethra, cervix, anus and throat and can occasionally infect the blood, joints and eyes.

How common is it and who gets it?

According to the Public Health Laboratory Service, there was an increase in cases in the 1960s and 1970s. Numbers fell sharply from 1985 but since 1994 cases have started to climb again and rose by 25 per cent between 1998 and 1999.

There were at least 16,500 cases in 1999 (many aren't detected because the infection is often symptomless). The latest figures show that new cases rose by 27 per cent between 1999 and 2000 to over 20,000. Key points about the figures are that about 40 per cent of the 6,223 diagnoses in women were in those aged 16 to 19. Men aged 20 to 24 are also at high risk, and diagnoses of gonorrhoea rose by 45 per cent between 1999 and 2000 in gay and bisexual men, an increase which is well above that for the general population.

What are the symptoms?

Symptoms will vary according to where in the body you've been infected. Symptoms can take 14 days to develop, although not everyone gets symptoms.

Women
- You may well not have any symptoms even if you are infected with gonorrhoea because as many as one in two women are symptomless.
- The commonest symptom is an increase or change in vaginal discharge, which may occur several days after infection. The discharge may change to a yellow or greenish colour and be smelly. Fewer than 10 per cent of women experience pelvic pain if the infection has moved upwards into the pelvis. You may find it difficult to pee if the urethra is infected, though you don't normally need to urinate more often. Gonorrhoea may occasionally cause bleeding between periods, or heavy periods.

Men
- Most common is a white, yellow or green discharge from the tip of the penis and a burning pain when peeing, sometimes inflammation of the testicles and a tender scrotum, possibly a discharge from the anus.
- Around 10 per cent of men with gonorrhoea have no symptoms.

Both sexes
An infection in the throat rarely causes symptoms but you may notice a sore throat. A rectal infection may cause pain and a discharge, but gonorrhoea is often symptomless – though gay men may be more prone to getting symptoms. Women can get anal infections even if they haven't had anal sex because secretions from an infected cervix can affect the anus.

How is it passed on?

Gonorrhoea is easily transmitted though unprotected vaginal, anal or oral sex – at least 5 per cent of cases are due to oral sex. It's more easily passed from men to women – for example, a woman who has unprotected sex with a man who's infected has around a 70 per cent chance of getting gonorrhoea. The risk of getting infected for a man who has unprotected sex with an infected woman is around 30 per cent.

It's much less common but the infection can be spread through rimming (where the tongue is used to stimulate the anus), or by finger contact; that is putting your fingers into an infected vagina, anus or mouth and then putting them into your own without washing your hands in between.

The infection can pass from mother to baby at birth causing conjunctivitis – inflammation of the lining of the eyes. About 30 per cent of babies born to infected mothers are affected.

Gonorrhoea can't be caught from towels or toilet seats.

Are there any complications?

It's important that gonorrhoea is treated as soon as possible because if it's not in about 10 per cent of women it can spread upwards into the pelvis where it can cause pelvic inflammatory disease. The result may be pelvic pain and painful sex as well as infertility or a potentially life-threatening ectopic pregnancy.

In men, the infection may also cause infertility in around 1 per cent of cases by causing inflammation and scarring in the epididymis.

It's rare, but untreated gonorrhoea may also cause other serious problems in men and women, such as an infection in the heart valves, or lining of the brain or spinal cord, or a blood infection, or joint problems.

How is it diagnosed?

Swabs are taken from the cervix in women and in both sexes from the urethra, and sometimes the throat and rectum. Tell the doctor what sort of sex you've had so swabs can be taken from all suspect areas. The bacteria can be looked for under the microscope to give a quick initial result, but are grown in the laboratory to confirm the diagnosis though this takes longer to do. A urine sample may also be taken.

What's the treatment?

- The aim is to clear the infection from all affected parts of the body. Gonorrhoea is treated with antibiotics, usually in tablet form though it can be by injection. About 95 per cent of cases are cured by a first dose of treatment – for example, a single 500mg tablet of ciprofloxacin or a single dose 400mg tablet of ofloxacin.
- Some strains of the bacteria are becoming increasingly resistant to some of the commonly used drugs but at the moment these drugs should normally be able to cure all straightforward cases of infection. If not there are alternatives – for example, a 250mg single injection of ceftriaxone.
- If you're pregnant, the normal drugs used to treat gonorrhoea aren't suitable so others such as ceftriaxone or amoxycillin may be used.
- If you've got a complicated infection, then longer antibiotic treatment will be needed.
- Up to 40 per cent of women and 20 per cent of men with gonorrhoea also have chlamydia so it's important also to be screened and treated for this.
- It's best not to have even protected sex during treatment. Check when you can safely have sex again.
- Even though your symptoms have gone it's important to see whether the treatment has worked. A test is normally done at least 72 hours after you've finished drug treatment – if you're infected

it may be that you've been reinfected rather than that the drugs haven't worked. If your throat was infected a throat swab is normally taken to check the infection has gone.

What about partners?

It's important that current and past partners over the last six months are tested in case they've got the infection. They'll be offered treatment, regardless of whether they're showing any signs of infection, to make sure they're not at risk.

Genital herpes

What is it?

Genital herpes is caused by the herpes simplex virus (HSV) which, according to the Herpes Viruses Association, is so common that three in four people will come into contact with it and carry it with or without symptoms.

Both types HSV1 and HSV2 can cause genital herpes or cold sores round the mouth (it used to be thought that HSV1 was responsible for cold sores and HSV2 for genital sores but it's now known that either type can cause genital sores or cold sores).

How common is it?

Genital herpes is very common and in 1999, 16,304 people were diagnosed as having a first attack of herpes. Figures have increased by 20 per cent for 2000 to 16,584. If you're aged 20 to 24 you're most at risk of getting it.

How do you get it?

- It's passed on through skin-to-skin contact so, for instance, you might get it from having sex with someone who has genital herpes or from oral sex if your partner has cold sores.
- A pregnant woman who has herpes may pass the virus to her baby during birth: if you developed genital herpes before getting pregnant there's a very low risk of passing it to your baby but if you get infected for the first time during pregnancy there's a bigger risk of passing it on – see the section on pregnancy.

- You can't catch herpes from toilet seats, from blood transfusions, from bath water or from towels.

How serious is it?

Genital herpes isn't serious, and it isn't linked to cervical cancer. Most people don't have significant problems with it. But there can be problems for your baby if you have a first attack when you're pregnant – see p. 63.

What are the symptoms?

Symptoms vary, and some people have none. But they may include the following:

- A tingling or itching feeling in the genital or anal area. Most commonly for men, around the penis, scrotum and urethra; and for women, on the lips of the vagina, and around the vagina, cervix and urethra. This is followed by small fluid blisters, which burst and leave small sores. These can be painful and may take a couple of weeks or so to heal. Also, there may be pain when you're urinating if the urine passes over any open sores. Flu-like symptoms with headaches, swollen glands and aching muscles.
- Symptoms may appear from four days after contact with the virus or may not appear for some weeks or months.
- Lots of people are unaware they've got herpes and only know about it when their partner develops symptoms.
- For some people a first attack can be quite severe and may take several weeks to heal.
- After the first attack the virus moves back from the skin deeper into the body but from time to time it may move back to the surface of the skin causing another attack, with perhaps an outbreak of symptoms.
- Some people get an early warning sign that the virus is becoming active again, what's called a 'prodrome'. You may notice your skin is more itchy, tingly or painful but you can't see anything on the skin.
- Recurrences are usually mild and don't happen very often. They may just last for around three days, though some people may get

more frequent severe recurrences, perhaps because their immune system isn't working very well.

How is herpes diagnosed?

It's possible that your symptoms could be confused with other conditions – for instance, an allergic reaction to soap or a spermicide or even cystitis if you're having pain when you urinate. It's estimated that only about one in five people are correctly diagnosed. To get an accurate diagnosis, a swab should be taken from the affected area to confirm that herpes is the cause of your problems – a diagnosis shouldn't be made just from the doctor examining you.

What's the treatment?

Genital herpes can't be cured with antibiotics because it's caused by a virus. Quick treatment of an attack with an antiviral drug may speed up healing time and how long you're affected, but won't stop recurrences.

Drug treatment for a first attack

Symptoms are usually worse with the first attack. If you're diagnosed quickly, within five days of infection, drugs such as aciclovir (200mg five times daily for around five days) can reduce the severity of symptoms. Tablets are better than creams unless you can't take the tablets because they make you vomit.

Other things that may help

The following remedies may also help or you can use them on their own if you haven't been diagnosed within five days of being infected or if you prefer not to take conventional antiviral treatment.

- Take painkillers such as ibuprofen or paracetamol (whatever works for you) for pain. Try an icepack on the affected area – wrap ice cubes or a pack of frozen peas in a flannel and place on the skin for a few minutes – never put the ice directly on the skin as it could damage it.
- Try gently bathing the sore area with a salt solution of one

61

teaspoon of salt to a pint of warm water. Use several times a day to help healing.
- Try using an anaesthetic such as lignocaine as a gel or ointment or in spray form on active sores to ease the pain. Ask your pharmacist what's available.

Recurrent infections

These are usually mild and you won't normally need drug treatment, though antiviral treatment taken continuously for a period of time can be used if you have severe and frequent attacks.

Self-help

These sorts of measures can help reduce recurrences.
- Take a multi-vitamin pill daily and have a varied, healthy diet with plenty of fresh fruit and vegetables.
- Bathe the genitals with cool water after exercise, sex or masturbation. Genital skin is delicate so use plenty of lubrication for sex to protect it.
- Wear loose-fitting, natural fibres round the genitals.
- Try to keep stress to a minimum, get enough sleep and try relaxation techniques such as yoga.
- Don't smoke, or cut down on it, and avoid too much alcohol.
  If you get early warning signs, the prodromal ones such as tingling, try the following: apply an icepack for 90 minutes – this may stop the sores developing and allow you some time to unwind.

Herbal help

- It is claimed that the herb melissa, commonly called 'lemon balm' can help prevent recurrence. In a trial, three-quarters of those using a cream containing lemon balm, Lomaherpan, found their genital sores didn't return when they were using it. The product is available from the Herpes Viruses Association (details at the end of the book).
- Olive leaf extract capsules taken daily may also be helpful as a preventative, according to the Association. For more details contact the Herpes Viruses Association.

How not to pass it on – partners

The risk of passing herpes on is greatest when the virus is active, but the problem is that you may not know when this is as lots of people have no symptoms. Condoms don't provide 100 per cent protection because they don't cover all affected skin.

It's a good idea to talk to a health adviser about the issues and about what you can do and how to discuss the fact that you've got herpes with a new partner. Normal advice is that it's best to do this before you become sexually intimate – you may find that your partner has genital herpes too.

Play safe. If you have genital or cold sores don't have genital or oral sex or kiss someone who is uninfected. Follow this rule from the first early warning signs if you get them through to when the sores are completely healed.

If you're sharing a bed at night, wear loose pyjamas or a nightie to lessen the risk of passing on the virus.

Pregnancy

Most women with herpes have no problems and have a normal pregnancy and a healthy baby. But there can be problems. A first attack during early pregnancy may result in miscarriage. A first attack during the last three months of pregnancy can mean the risk of passing it to your baby may be 50 per cent, and babies can be seriously affected by herpes. If you develop herpes before getting pregnant this problem shouldn't arise because antibodies in your body will give protection to your baby.

- As a general precaution, let your doctor or midwife know if you or your partner has ever had herpes and let them know if you get a first attack of herpes during pregnancy.
- Ideally before you get pregnant talk to your doctor about your options if your partner has genital herpes but you've never had herpes symptoms.
- If you're pregnant and want to know what your risks are, you may be advised to get tested for herpes. If you don't have antibodies to the virus it's important to try to avoid getting an attack for the first time during pregnancy. General advice would be not to have sex if your partner has genital sores or cold sores and to use condoms at

63

all times to reduce risk. Some doctors might even say you should avoid all sexual contact for the rest of the pregnancy if you have no antibodies to the infection.

Herpes management during pregnancy

First attacks

If you become infected for the first time during the first six months of pregnancy, your doctor may advise antiviral drug treatment then and also in the last four weeks of pregnancy so that you don't need to have a Caesarean. If you become infected during the last three months your doctor will discuss the pros and cons of having a Caesarean, particularly if you're within six weeks of the birth, in order to protect the baby. If you have a vaginal delivery then the doctor may advise antiviral treatment for both you and the baby.

Recurrent attacks

If you develop herpes before you became pregnant and get recurrent attacks during pregnancy you're unlikely to have problems but there's a very small risk of passing it to your baby if you get an attack near to delivery. You shouldn't normally need a Caesarean if you don't have genital sores at the time of birth, but if you do have sores just before the birth a Caesarean may be suggested, though the pros and cons of this need to be discussed with you.

5

Bacterial Vaginosis, Cystitis and Thrush

I've put these three common conditions in a chapter of their own. They're not sexually transmitted infections but they're common among people who're sexually active.

Bacterial vaginosis

What is it and who gets it?

Bacterial vaginosis (BV) is the commonest cause of abnormal vaginal discharge in women of childbearing age and results from a change in the bacterial balance in the vagina. The main type of bacteria in the vagina are lactobacilli, which keep the vagina slightly acidic and healthy.

For various reasons that aren't fully understood, the bacterial balance changes are associated with BV and the vagina becomes more alkaline as potentially harmful organisms known as 'anaerobic bacteria' flourish, increasing by as much as a thousand times. They don't need oxygen and include organisms like *Gardnerella vaginalis, Mycoplasma hominis.*

According to specialists in genito-urinary medicine, BV is more common in black than white women, in women who have an IUD fitted and in those who smoke.

BV is not regarded as an STI and you don't need to be sexually active to have it; on the other hand it seems mainly to affect women who regularly have sex. It's also more common among lesbians, according to one study, which found that 33 per cent of lesbians had BV compared to 13 per cent of non-lesbians.

Although BV is not an STI, about 18 per cent of women with it also have chlamydia. It's not understood why this should happen but it may be that a chlamydial infection triggers changes in the vaginal environment, which allow the oxygen-hating bacteria to grow.

BV is a puzzling condition and nobody knows for sure at the moment why it develops. Things that may play a part include:

hormonal changes, infections such as chlamydia, excessive washing of the genitals and douching (washing out the vagina), perfumed soap, also smoking and having an IUD.

How common is it?

BV is very common. Estimates vary from one in three women to one in five or one in ten who will get it at some point in their lives. In 1999, 59,435 cases were reported at sexual health clinics in the UK.

What are the symptoms?

- Fifty per cent of women are symptomless.
- When they occur, symptoms are mild and include a distinctive fishy-smelling vaginal discharge, which smells more after sex and during periods. The discharge may increase, become thin and watery and change to a white/grey colour. The discharge doesn't normally cause itching, soreness or irritation but it may be misdiagnosed as thrush even though this itches a lot – see the section on thrush (pp. 71–4).

Are there any complications?

BV used to be thought of as a harmless condition but there's increasing evidence that women who have BV in early pregnancy have a much higher risk – fivefold – of late miscarriage between 16 and 24 weeks, or an increased risk of having a baby born prematurely between 24 and 27 weeks. BV may also be linked to infection after gynaecological procedures such as hysterectomy, abortion and possibly IUD insertion, as well as to pelvic inflammatory disease.

How is it diagnosed?

A vaginal swab is taken and several things analysed: the type of discharge, what sorts of cells are in the discharge, and the acidity of the discharge. Also its smell: a chemical called potassium hydroxide is added to the sample which produces a characteristic fishy smell if you have BV.

It's a good idea to ask about getting tested if you suspect you have BV and are going to have some sort of gynaecological procedure or if you want to get pregnant – see the section on pregnancy on p. 68.

What's the treatment?

The aim of treatment is to allow the normal vaginal bacteria to return so that the lactobacilli flourish again. A drug is used to kill off the oxygen-hating bacteria and the usual treatment is with the antibiotic metronidazole (Flagyl) which is highly effective and has a 80 to 90 per cent success rate. It's usually taken for five to seven days, 400 to 500mg twice daily as a tablet; or as a single 2g dose; or as a vaginal gel for five days. You shouldn't drink alcohol when you take the treatment in tablet form as this will make you feel very ill and you'll get severe nausea and vomiting; if you're using the vaginal gel also avoid alcohol. A nasty taste in the mouth after taking the pill should go if you have a glass of water.

An alternative is another antibiotic – clindamycin – used internally as a vaginal cream for seven days. Clindamycin cream may weaken rubber condoms and diaphragms so you may be advised to use plastic products instead to protect yourself against infections and pregnancy.

Check whether you can have sex during treatment – if you have other infections then you'll be advised against this.

If you're breastfeeding and need treatment then you should normally be given a vaginal cream rather than tablets, as small amounts of the drug can get into breast milk.

Though treatment works well, BV often recurs. Some women try to treat themselves by buying lactic acid products – available from the pharmacy without prescription – which aim to make the vagina more acidic. But bear in mind that these preparations won't cure BV and you could be at risk of getting the sorts of problems discussed above; for instance in pregnancy or after gynaecological procedures.

Partners

- There's no evidence that male partners need to be treated, but since women with BV often have chlamydia too it's a good idea for both men and women to be tested for infections generally.
- BV may be more common in lesbians, as I've said, and if you're being treated for BV, ask whether it's a good idea for your partner to be treated. It's possible that BV could be passed between women through sex toys contaminated with vaginal fluid so wash the toy between usages or put a new condom on it.

What about pregnancy?

If you want to get pregnant, talk to your doctor about whether you should be checked for BV infection. Research suggests screening may be a good idea if you've previously given birth early for no obvious reason or lost your baby in the second three months of pregnancy. Some specialists advocate routine screening of all pregnant women in early pregnancy. If treatment is needed because of a positive result discuss your treatment options with your doctor. Advice at the moment is that you should be retested a month later and treated again if BV has come back.

Prevention

Though it's not clear at the moment what triggers BV, it's worth trying these things. Don't douche, or use vaginal deodorants or bubble baths. Don't use perfumed soaps and try using an aqueous cream in preference to non-perfumed soap. If you're fitted with an IUD, talk to your doctor about whether you should try some other contraceptive method.

Some women eat live yoghurt or insert it in the vagina, or take lactobacilli supplements to try to keep the vaginal bacteria in balance, but it's not clear how well these measures work.

Cystitis

What is it?

The strict medical definition is inflammation of the bladder lining, most often caused by a bacterial infection – about 80 per cent of cases are thought to be caused by *E. coli* bacteria from the bowel. Sometimes the infection can move upwards from the bladder to the kidneys, causing more serious problems.

There's a lot of confusion about the term 'cystitis' because people often use the term to describe urethritis, symptoms caused by an inflamed urethra, the tube from the bladder through which urine is passed. (Interstitial cystitis is much less common, affecting about one in 400 women with bladder problems, and is a chronic type of cystitis in which the bladder lining is inflamed but there's no obvious bacterial infection.)

Who gets cystitis?

Men can get cystitis but women are much more prone to it because the entrance to the urethra is very close to the vagina and anus and a woman's urethra is very short compared to a man's. All of which means that organisms from the vagina and anus can easily irritate the urethra and the short urethra makes it easier for the bladder to become infected. The rest of this section on cystitis is written for women. Men's urethral problems are looked at in the section on non-specific urethritis (see pp. 87–90).

What are the symptoms?

Pain when you urinate, an urgent need to urinate even when there's no urine to pass, sometimes blood in the urine, fever, and backache if the kidneys are infected.

What causes it?

Cystitis is not an STI and you don't catch it. As we've seen, the strict definition of cystitis is inflammation of the bladder lining most often caused by a bacterial infection such as *E. coli* but there are other things that can irritate the urethra: irritants such as perfumed soap and bath oils, bruising of the urethra during sex – that's why cystitis is sometimes called 'honeymoon cystitis'. Vaginal infections such as thrush can irritate the urethra, as can STIs such as chlamydia; spermicides and rubber diaphragms may cause problems in some women.

How is it diagnosed?

The only way to check for bacterial infection in the urine is to have a midstream urine sample taken, which can be sent off to the laboratory for analysis. If cystitis keeps coming back a cystoscopy may be done in which a special viewing instrument is passed through the urethra to look at the inside of the bladder. Ask your doctor about whether you should have a test for diabetes if you keep getting attacks and have a family history of diabetes. Diabetic women are more prone to attacks because extra sugar in the vagina can make them more prone to thrush, which in turn may cause cystitis-type symptoms.

If you think you or your partner could have an STI, go to a sexual health clinic.

What's the treatment?

Many attacks can be successfully self-managed. At the first twinges, take a dose of a painkiller and drink lots of water – half a pint of water every 20 minutes for three hours. You can buy products such as Cymalon, which are available without a prescription from the pharmacy. These contain substances such as potassium citrate that alkalinize the urine, making it more comfortable to pass.

When to see the doctor

If your symptoms don't start to improve after 24 hours or if they worsen, see your doctor; particularly if you feel feverish, have blood in your urine or a low backache, in case the infection has moved upwards into your kidneys.

A urine sample will normally be taken. At the moment doctors normally prescribe a three-day course of antibiotics such as trimethoprim straight away rather than waiting to get the results of the urine sample, which may take several days to come back from the laboratory. But another antibiotic may be needed if the urine results reveal an antibiotic-resistant bacterium.

Prevention

There are lots of things you can do to prevent a cystitis attack:

- Keep the crotch airy by wearing cotton briefs, don't use perfumed soaps and oils in the bath, drink plenty of fluids to flush germs out of your bladder and to stop urine becoming too acidic (acidic urine is more uncomfortable to pass).
- Sex: wash your genitals beforehand and your partner should wash theirs, too; use lots of non-irritant lubricants before penetration to stop damage to delicate tissue; spermicides, badly fitting diaphragms and rubber condoms can sometimes cause problems – solutions include: using plastic condoms as these shouldn't cause an allergic reaction; avoiding spermicides or finding if there's one that doesn't irritate you; getting the diaphragm properly fitted; emptying your bladder immediately after sex to flush out any germs.

• Practise safer sex.

Thrush

What is it?

Thrush is a yeast infection caused by the fungus *Candida albicans*; the medical name is 'candidiasis' or 'candidosis' but the infection is commonly called 'thrush' or candida. This fungus lives in the body – for instance, in the mouth, gut and vagina, where it usually causes no problems and is kept in check by good bacteria but for a number of reasons the fungus can get out of balance, causing problems in the vagina and the penis.

How common is it?

It's very common, and in 1999 over 70,000 cases of genital candidosis were reported at STI clinics. Men can get it in the penis, particularly if they're not circumcised, but it's vaginal thrush that is so common; one estimate is that three out of four women will get it at some point in their lives.

Is thrush an STI?

You don't have to be sexually active to get thrush but it's very common in sexually active people, and you may get it if you have sex with someone who has thrush though you don't normally catch it as such from other people. Sex is more likely to play a role if it damages delicate vaginal tissues as this can sometimes trigger an attack.

Is it serious?

No, but it can make your life a misery if you keep getting it.

What causes thrush?

It can occur for various reasons.

• Antibiotics (e.g. for other infection) may destroy beneficial bacteria in the vagina, allowing the fungus to multiply.
• Tight synthetic clothes around the crotch may encourage it because the yeast loves warm moist areas.
• The yeast is often in the digestive tract and may be carried from the bowel to the vagina.

71

- If you're in poor health or under a lot of stress your immune system won't be so able to fight off a thrush infection. If you're prescribed certain drugs such as steroids you may also be more prone to getting thrush.
- Diabetes that isn't properly controlled may make you more susceptible to getting thrush because high sugar levels in the blood could reduce vaginal acidity, making it more likely that the fungus gets out of control.
- An allergic reaction to a spermicide may allow the fungus to overgrow.
- Hormonal changes during pregnancy, just before a period or if you're on the contraceptive pill may trigger thrush.
- Damage to delicate genital tissues during sex can cause thrush.

What are the symptoms?

Women

The most common symptom of thrush is intense itching around the vagina, which can be very embarrassing. There may be soreness in and around the vagina if tissue is inflamed. Vaginal discharge may be heavier and thicker than usual, a bit like cottage cheese but it doesn't usually smell. If the vagina is inflamed, sex may be painful; and peeing may be uncomfortable as urine stings the inflamed tissues round the vagina – the urinary symptoms may sometimes be confused with those of cystitis.

Men

Symptoms include irritation, burning and itching under the foreskin on the tip of the penis, possibly red patches there, a thick discharge under the foreskin, discomfort when peeing (after unprotected sex you may notice a burning sensation, which often disappears after you've had a shower).

How is it diagnosed?

If you think you have thrush and you've never had it before, see your doctor or go to a clinic. Don't self-diagnose and treat it in case it's something else.

As well as looking for signs of infection, a swab is taken from the vagina in women and from under the foreskin in men.

Whats the treatment?

Antifungal drugs that work throughout the body can be taken, or creams and pessaries can be used where the problem is. Many of these are available over the counter from the pharmacy – for example, fluconazole (Diflucan One) or Canesten Once.

As I've said, symptoms of thrush may be confused with other conditions such as cystitis, so with a first attack it's important to see your doctor to get a proper diagnosis. Make sure to say if you're pregnant because you shouldn't take fluconazole, for instance, if you're pregnant.

It's a good idea not to have sex while you're getting better and you probably won't want to because you're too uncomfortable. Don't scratch yourself and don't wash with very hot water. Pat yourself dry gently with a clean towel when you're washing yourself. At the first sign of problems, if you can't get to a doctor or pharmacist, try washing in a diluted salt solution one teaspoon of table salt dissolved in a pint of warm water. Some women find that live yoghurt applied on a tampon eases the itching and may sometimes ward off an attack.

Recurrent thrush

Some people keep on getting thrush attacks. A recent study reported that women who do should have longer drug treatment with tablets and then further preventive treatment at regular intervals, say using a pessary (a medicated plug that's inserted into the vagina) once or twice a month. Research carried out on 120 women found that after initial treatment the same yeast strain was responsible for later attacks. The women seemed to have persistent infections rather than be reinfected or to have an infection that was resistant to the antifungal treatment.

Get checked for diabetes in case this is the underlying reason for your thrush.

Partners

Make sure your partner is treated to avoid reinfection. Men don't always have symptoms so if you keep getting thrush it's a good idea for them to be checked even if they don't have obvious symptoms or signs.

Prevention

- During sex, protect genital tissue by making sure you're properly lubricated.
- Avoid bubble baths which can kill off protective bacteria, and avoid using perfumed soaps on the genitals. Use unperfumed soaps or soap replacement products, such as aqueous cream, which clean more gently. Don't douche.
- Tampons can sometimes aggravate thrush so if you use these try pads instead.
- The yeast thrives in moist, warm conditions so avoid tights and wear loose-fitting skirts and trousers.
- Boost your immune system by eating a diet rich in fruit and vegetables and cut back on foods containing yeast (e.g. bread, blue cheese, mushrooms) and reduce the amount of sugar you eat.
- Try eating live yoghurt each day.
- You may be more prone to thrush if you're anaemic, so have a blood test done if you think this could be the case (e.g. you have heavy periods and feel tired all the time).
- Wipe from front to back after a bowel movement.
- Some contraceptive pills may make you more susceptible to getting thrush so talk to your doctor about whether you should change to a different pill or try another contraceptive method.
- Steroids suppress the immune system and can make you more vulnerable to thrush, so if you're on them long term and keep getting thrush, talk to your doctor about what your options are (e.g. whether your steroid treatment can be altered in any way).

6

HIV and Hepatitis

HIV

Human immunodeficiency virus (HIV) is not the commonest of STIs but it's the one most people know about. It's a life-threatening infection which came to light in the 1980s.

What is it?

It's a virus, which, because it weakens the immune system, the body's defence system, results eventually in serious illness. To become infected, enough HIV must get into your bloodstream. The virus isn't that infectious compared to some other infections.

Body fluids that contain sufficient HIV to infect you are blood, sperm and seminal fluid, vaginal fluids including menstrual fluids and breast milk. But saliva, urine and sweat don't contain enough HIV to cause infection, according to the Terrence Higgins Trust, the UK's leading HIV and AIDS charity.

How do you get it?

You don't get HIV through the air, as with the cold virus. For HIV to be transmitted there needs to be infected body fluids, and these fluids have to get into the bloodstream.

There are several ways of getting the virus but the commonest one is having unprotected vaginal or anal sex with someone who is infected. For women, HIV may pass through the vagina, the cervix or the urethra; and for men through the urethra; and the virus can also pass through the rectum in both men and women.

Oral sex
- HIV can be passed on through oral sex. Advice from the Public Health Laboratory Service in 2001 says there's a much smaller risk of getting HIV from oral sex than from unprotected anal and vaginal sex – unprotected anal sex is most risky, responsible for over 90 per cent of HIV cases in gay men. But though oral sex is much less risky, it may be responsible for more infections than

was previously thought. At the moment oral sex may account for between 3 and 8 per cent of HIV infections in gay men.

Sucking the penis of a man with HIV is the type of oral sex most likely to lead to the passing on of the virus and, in most cases when this has happened, it's been through sores or cuts in the person's mouth.

Less risky is licking the genitals of a woman who has HIV because there's much less of the virus in vaginal fluid; though the risk could be higher if she's got her period because more of the virus is present in menstrual blood. It's also possible but less likely that the virus can be passed on if the person sucking or licking has HIV, particularly if the person receiving oral sex has cuts in the genitals, such as piercings in the penis or vaginal area that haven't healed completely.

- Shared sex toys, where the toy is put into the vagina or anus, can be a source of transmission from one person to another if the sex toy isn't washed or doesn't have a clean condom put on it between users.
- A mother can pass the virus to her baby during pregnancy and birth and when breastfeeding.
- HIV can also be picked up from a blood transfusion, though since 1985 blood and tissue donations have been tested for HIV in the UK. Infected blood products can pass on HIV – for instance, the blood given to haemophiliacs – but blood products are treated now to destroy any HIV that might be present.
- Sharing drug-injecting equipment with someone who is infected (5.5 per cent of those infected in 1998 got it this way) can pass on HIV.
- Sharing toothbrushes and razors, and having any procedure which pierces the skin (e.g. acupuncture or tattooing) could theoretically be risky though there aren't thought to be any recorded cases of people getting HIV this way.

How common is HIV?

HIV is most widespread in the continents of Africa and Asia; proportionally far fewer people in the UK are infected. But the Department of Health says there's no room for complacency. In 2000 there were 3,435 new cases of HIV, 14 per cent more than in

1999, the highest number of new cases in a year since testing became widely available in the UK in 1985. Sex between men is still the main way that the virus is passed on, although there's been an increase in HIV for heterosexuals, perhaps because people are more prepared to be tested now. The virus has also significantly affected communities in the UK from those parts of Africa where HIV has a stronghold.

Who gets it?

According to the Terrence Higgins Trust, people at particular risk are:

- gay men – 56 per cent of men in 1998 became infected through unprotected sex with other men;
- men and women who inject drugs plus their sexual partners.

Getting tested

The only way to find out whether you've got HIV is to be tested. The commonest sort of test is a blood test, which looks for antibodies to the virus produced by the immune system, but it needs to be done three months after you've been infected. If it's done earlier your body may not yet have produced enough antibodies to show up in the test. This three-month period is called the 'window period' or 'seroconversion'. If antibodies are found, it means you're infected and are HIV-positive. If you test negative then you don't have HIV, provided the test was done at the right time and not too soon after you'd been exposed to the virus.

Another test that may be done sometimes but isn't routinely offered is a blood test that looks for a part of the virus that can be detected. This can be done around two to three weeks after infection.

The Department of Health wants HIV testing to be offered routinely in all sexual health clinics. At the moment it's offered to all pregnant women as part of their antenatal care.

What happens if you have HIV?

For a time your immune system can usually keep the virus in check but the virus damages the immune system, especially white blood cells known as 'CD4 cells', and eventually over time the number of healthy CD4 cells decline and the amount of virus increases. The result is that your immune system can't fight infections so well.

You may feel fine for a number of years, though some people may experience short periods of illness, such as sore throat, fever or a rash when the body starts to produce antibodies to the virus.

As the virus increases in the body, the immune system becomes less able to work properly, which means you may become more vulnerable to infections that wouldn't normally be troublesome if your immune system was working at full strength.

Early signs that the immune system isn't working so well include developing or worsening of skin problems such as psoriasis, or other problems such as thrush in the mouth, fevers and shingles.

AIDS (acquired immune deficiency syndrome) means your immune system has got to a point where it can't cope and when what are called 'opportunistic infections' develop. Examples of these are: a rare form of pneumonia, certain types of cancers, severe cytomegalovirus infections, and toxoplasmosis.

What's the treatment?

Levels of the virus in your blood and your CD4 count are monitored.

There's still no cure for HIV but things have changed. In the past most HIV-positive people developed AIDS but this doesn't happen to the same extent now. Early treatment using highly active anti-retroviral drug therapy – HAART for short – can delay the development of AIDs by slowing down the damaging effects of HIV. After the introduction of HAART in 1996, AIDS cases dropped from 1,024 for that year to 478 cases in 2000.

The treatment doesn't destroy the virus and isn't a magic bullet, but it does suppress the virus. HAART isn't straightforward. Treatment may not work so well if you don't maintain a certain level of drugs in the body. The drugs are complicated and need to be taken in the right way, at the right time and in precise doses for best effect, and the drugs may have side-effects.

It's not clear at the moment whether combination therapy can work indefinitely and it may also not work if the virus becomes resistant to the drugs. A trial is taking place to see whether it's better to take five instead of the three drugs used at the moment.

In addition to the antiviral drugs, antibiotics may be needed to protect you against opportunistic infections such as toxoplasmosis.

Prevention

There's no vaccination for HIV at the moment.

Practise safer sex and use condoms (remember that even if both of you are HIV-negative or -positive, you still need protection against other STIs).

It's possible but difficult for HIV to be passed on through oral sex. The most likely sort of oral sex that could lead to HIV infection is sucking the penis of an infected man – there's virus in the semen but it's difficult for the virus to survive in your mouth and get from there into the bloodstream. But this could be easier if your partner comes off in your mouth and you have cuts and sores or gum disease in your mouth. You're also more at risk of HIV if you have gonorrhoea in your throat as this damages skin, which again makes it easier for HIV to get into the bloodstream.

Risks can be reduced by the man not coming in his partner's mouth, though pre-ejaculate can still transmit the virus. The best way to reduce risks is by using a condom.

Keep your mouth healthy because the virus can pass more easily through damaged tissue. Don't brush or floss just before oral sex, especially if your gums bleed, and don't use a mouthwash just before or after oral sex as it may remove protective substances in saliva. Recent dental surgery may also increase the risk of transmission so be particularly careful if you've had this – it's probably best to avoid oral sex until your mouth has completely healed.

- Anal–oral sex is low risk for HIV though of course other infections can be passed this way.
- The skin acts as a barrier to infection so keep it healthy and use lots of lubrication for sex.
- Sexual activities that carry very little risk of HIV infection are kissing, body-rubbing, fingering and mutual masturbation.
- If you're going abroad to places such as sub-Saharan Africa, Asia, Eastern Europe, Spain and Italy, or having sex with someone from those countries where HIV infection is more prevalent than in the UK, it's particularly important to have protected sex. If you're going abroad take good-quality condoms with you.
- Don't share needles.

Pregnancy

The virus can be passed from a mother to her baby but steps can be taken to stop this happening. HIV-positive mums are given a short course of an anti-HIV drug a few weeks before birth and drug treatment continues for both mum and baby for a short time after the birth; babies are delivered by Caesarean; breastfeeding should be avoided. These three measures can reduce the risk of the baby of an infected mum getting HIV to about two in 100.

In 1999 the Department of Health offered and recommended HIV testing to all pregnant women as part of their standard pregnancy tests. As a result, 73 per cent of pregnant women had their infection diagnosed before delivery which meant that the steps mentioned above could be taken to protect the baby.

Partners

You'll be counselled about partners who may be at risk and need to be traced.

Hepatitis

Hepatitis means inflammation of the liver which can be caused by various things like alcohol, some drugs and some viruses. Three viruses are looked at below which can be passed on in various ways including through sex.

Hepatitis A

Hepatitis A is found in contaminated food and water but is also found in faeces – shit – and you can get infected if your mouth comes into contact with faeces, even a tiny amount, from someone who has the virus. This means it can be passed on if you're having sex that brings you into contact with faeces. For example, if you stimulate your partner's anus with your tongue (called 'rimming' or 'analingus'), or if you put your fingers in your partner's anus, don't wash them and then put them in your mouth. Hepatitis is common among gay men but anyone who does rimming needs to know about this risk.

What are the symptoms?

There may not be any symptoms of hepatitis A, or they may be so mild you don't notice them. Several weeks after infection you may have flu-like symptoms, fever, diarrhoea, feeling tired and sick, having itchy skin, loss of appetite, weight loss, the whites of the eyes may turn yellow. Whether or not you have symptoms, you can still pass on the virus and are most infectious before symptoms show.

How is hepatitis A diagnosed?
A blood test is needed. It may show you've had a past infection and now have natural protection against future infection with the virus. If the results are negative it means you haven't been in contact with the virus and have no natural protection against it.

What's the treatment?
Infection is usually mild but occasionally you may get severe liver inflammation in which case you'll need treatment. Rest is important, and while your liver recovers you shouldn't drink alcohol because the liver has to process this. Check with your doctor but avoid any medicines that may stress the liver. Recovery can take about three months.

Partners
The clinic will advise about who should be contacted.

Prevention
- General hygiene is important so always wash your hands after going to the toilet. If you practise rimming, use a latex barrier between your mouth and your partner's anus; wash your hands carefully after disposing of used condoms, or touching sex toys or your partner's anus.
- Get vaccinated against hepatitis A. Ask what's available at the sexual health clinic. You may be offered an immunoglobulin vaccination (an injection of antibodies). There are two types of vaccination. The first is short term and provides protection against the virus for a few months. The second type (which may be the vaccination of choice if you're gay) is given as two injections; the

first injection provides protection for a year and the second is effective for ten more years. After that a booster is needed. Before having the vaccination a blood test will show if you have antibodies against the virus, in which case you won't need the vaccination.

Hepatitis B

Hepatitis B is very common and very infectious and is found in body fluids, including blood, saliva, semen and vaginal fluid. It's passed on in various ways – sex, sharing contaminated drug needles, non-sterilized equipment being used for things like acupuncture, tattooing or body-piercing, from an infected mother to her baby, through blood transfusions where the blood hasn't been tested for the virus. In the UK all donated blood is tested for hepatitis B.

The two commonest ways in which hepatitis B is passed on are through using contaminated needles to inject drugs and through sexual contact. It can be passed on easily through unprotected penetrative anal, vaginal or oral sex. The virus is also present in saliva so it's possible it could be passed on by kissing though this isn't common. Hepatitis B is common among gay and bisexual men but also among people who have lots of partners.

What are the symptoms of hepatitis B?

You may not notice any, or you may get flu-like symptoms, feel tired, exhausted and nauseous, develop diarrhoea, lose your appetite, lose weight, the whites of the eyes and skin may go yellow, you may develop itchy skin. Symptoms usually appear one to four months after infection.

Most people get over their symptoms and stop being infectious, but up to 10 per cent of people who get infected with the virus feel healthy but are carriers and infectious to others, though some get rid of the virus after some years. Around 30 per cent of carriers may develop chronic liver damage and over a number of years risk getting liver cancer and other liver problems such as cirrhosis, when liver tissue becomes abnormal. Infected newborn babies are also more at risk of becoming carriers and developing severe liver problems later in life.

A few people with hepatitis B also have hepatitis D – the D virus needs the B virus to survive and if you have the two viruses you're more at risk of getting serious liver disease.

How is it diagnosed?

Hepatitis B is diagnosed by a blood test that looks for antibodies produced by the body in response to the virus or for particles of the virus itself. The tests can show various things – for instance, whether you have been infected and cleared the infection or whether you're a carrier.

What's the treatment?

Often no treatment is needed but it's important to rest, avoid alcohol or anything that stresses the liver, and avoid fatty food. Antiviral medicine – interferon – may be used to control the virus if you have a chronic infection.

Partners

The clinic will advise on who should be contacted, tested and immunized if necessary.

Prevention

- Practise safer sex.
- Vaccination: if you're at high risk (gays, bisexuals or heterosexuals who have many sexual partners) you should get vaccinated. Sexual health clinics give the vaccination so discuss your options there. The Department of Health's National Sexual Health Strategy document sets out various targets for vaccination and in particular says that by the end of 2003 all gay and bisexual men attending sexual health clinics should be offered vaccination on their first visit. Three injections are given over 3 to 6 months, and the protection should last for at least five years. If you know your partner is infected, ask about vaccination. If you have been exposed to the virus, you should get an injection of antibodies called 'immunoglobulin' to give you short-term protection plus the vaccination.

Pregnancy

If you contract hepatitis B during the last three months of pregnancy there's a very good chance that the infection will be passed on to your baby. Since 2000 all pregnant women in the UK are tested for the virus. If a woman is infected, her baby is given an immunoglobulin injection immediately after birth to stop the baby becoming infected.

Hepatitis C

Hepatitis C hasn't been known about for long but it's common and can be very serious.

How can you get it?

- The virus is mainly in blood and you're most at risk of getting infected if you share contaminated needles or other drug-injecting equipment.
- It can be spread through blood transfusions in countries where blood isn't tested for the virus; blood is tested in the UK.
- It's not passed on as easily as hepatitis B through sex. It's thought that about 5 per cent of people get hepatitis C by sexual contact through unprotected anal or vaginal sex because semen and vaginal secretions contain enough of the virus to pass it on. But this figure could be higher and it may turn out that sex plays a bigger role in transmission. A third of cases of hepatitis C have no known cause and it could be that sex played a role in some of these cases. People with lots of sexual partners also run a higher risk of getting infected. It's unlikely to be passed on through oral sex unless there's bleeding from the penis or mouth. If you've got sores in the genital area (e.g. genital herpes) it may be easier to get hepatitis C.
- Occasionally an infected mother can pass the virus to her baby during labour and there's a greater risk of this happening if she has HIV.

What are the symptoms?

Many people don't notice any symptoms when they're first infected but they can still pass the hepatitis C virus on. Symptoms, when they occur – usually one to two months after infection – include a mild flu-like illness, nausea, vomiting, diarrhoea, weight loss, yellow skin and whites of the eyes, dark yellow urine, and itchy skin.

What happens if you're infected?

There's much that's not understood about how the virus affects people. It's thought that about one in five infected people seems to clear the virus from the blood but four or five remain infected and over time – perhaps years – may develop liver problems, such as liver cancer, chronic inflammation of the liver, and cirrhosis of the liver where liver tissue becomes abnormal and the liver can't function properly.

What's the test?

You'll be given a test for antibodies to the virus and if this is positive it means you've been exposed to the virus at some point, but it doesn't show whether you've still got the virus or whether you're infectious. If the test is done too soon after exposure to the virus, the result may show up as negative. Another blood test may be done to look for the virus itself.

What's the treatment?

If you've got an active infection, you'll be monitored by a liver specialist and tests will be done to see how well your liver is working. You need to be very careful about how much alcohol you drink and to avoid fatty foods. Drugs such as interferon are used to halt and slow the disease process sometimes together with a man-made drug called 'ribavirin'. There are various strains of hepatitis C and some strains are more resistant to drug treatment so you'll be tested to see which one you have before treatment.

Partners

The clinic should advise you about who needs to be notified. Ask what you should do to protect your partner if you're in a long-term relationship.

Prevention

At the moment you can't be vaccinated against the hepatitis C virus. Always use condoms during sex and plenty of lubricants, particularly for anal sex, to reduce the risk of bleeding, which increases the chances of the virus being transmitted. Don't share things like toothbrushes and razors with someone who is infected, and don't share drug-injecting equipment.

7

Infections from M to T

Molluscum contagiosum

What is it, how common is it and how do you get it?

Molluscum contagiosum is caused by a virus and it's common; there were 8,065 cases in 1999 at sexual health clinics in the UK but lots of people don't seek treatment for this harmless skin condition so this figure doesn't reflect the true number of cases.

It's passed through close physical contact, which doesn't have to be sexual so children often get it but adults can also be infected through sexual contact.

What are the symptoms?

The virus causes small bumps or spots on the skin that are called 'papules'. They are usually flesh-coloured but can also be white, yellow or pink. However, not everyone gets symptoms. The 'bumps' as they're often called don't normally itch or hurt. They have a characteristic dent in the middle, which can be hard to see with the naked eye. If you squeeze it you get a bit of fluid, which contains the virus.

The bumps normally appear about one week to several months after you're infected but can take much longer to appear in some people. The bumps may appear on their own or in groups, and in various places on the body. When sexually transmitted, they may occur on the thighs and on the genitals and on the outside skin rather than internally. The spots are sometimes confused with warts.

What happens?

Left untreated, the bumps usually heal and disappear and don't leave any scars. This can happen quickly within about one week but can also take much longer, up to four years.

Are there any complications?

If your immune system is working properly there aren't any problems but if, for instance, you have HIV the bumps of *Molluscum contagiosum* may appear in less usual places such as the face and neck and can be very large.

How is it diagnosed?

The appearance of the bumps is characteristic; the spots are normally less than 2mm in size. There's no blood test used for diagnosis.

What about pregnancy?

The bumps don't pose any risks to your baby if you get them when you're pregnant.

Is there any treatment?

Since the spots usually disappear on their own, no treatment is needed. But the most commonly used treatment if you want to get rid of them before they go of their own accord includes freezing, though this may leave scars, so you need to discuss whether it's a good idea to have this. Another practical way of dealing with the spots is to press them to remove the liquid containing the core of the virus. Another option is to consult a medical herbalist to see if herbal treatment can help to remove the spots more quickly (see details for the National Institute of Medical Herbalists in Chapter 8).

If the spots are red, tender and filled with pus then they may be infected with a common bacteria found on the skin, such as staphylococcus, in which case you may need antibiotic treatment.

Partners

It's best to avoid sexual contact until the spots have cleared though this isn't essential – for more advice talk to a health adviser. If your partner doesn't have symptoms there's no need for treatment but if they do it's a good idea for the diagnosis to be confirmed by a clinic.

Non-specific urethritis

What is it?

Non-specific urethritis (NSU) is a condition that occurs in men. Also called 'non-gonococcal urethritis' (i.e. it's not caused by gonorrhoea), it's a catch-all term used to describe inflammation of the urethra, the tube which carries urine from the bladder to the tip of the penis. The term was first used at a time when few laboratory tests were available to detect organisms and it just wasn't clear what organisms were responsible for symptoms.

Women too can get urethral problems; for instance, as discussed in the sections on chlamydia and cystitis, but NSU is normally used to describe urethral problems in men. NSU is a common problem and in 1999, 58,528 cases were reported at clinics in the UK.

How do you get it?

- The commonest cause is sexual infection through unprotected vaginal, anal or oral sex.
- Chlamydia is the commonest cause of urethral inflammation, accounting for 30 to 50 per cent of cases. In the past, tests might not have detected this and men would have been told they had NSU though it wasn't clear what was causing the problem.
- Less frequently other STIs, such as *Trichomonas vaginalis* (discussed later in this chapter) and types of candida, also the herpes simplex virus.
- Vigorous sexual activity may damage the urethra.
- Bladder infection.
- Allergy to bubble baths or washing powders.
- May possibly be linked in some way to a vaginal infection in their partner, such as bacterial vaginosis.
- In about 30 per cent of men, no NSU organism can be detected, though this doesn't mean there isn't one; just that it can't be detected at the moment with present technology.

What are the symptoms?

- Discharge from the tip of the penis, pain when urinating and an increased need to urinate.
- Some men have no symptoms.

Are there any complications?

For a small number of men, perhaps fewer than 1 per cent, complications may occur, such as inflammation of the epididymis or prostate, infertility or Reiter's syndrome which may cause inflammation of the eyes, joints and urethra.

How is it diagnosed?

The genitals are examined and a swab taken from the urethra for analysis to look for various organisms. A urine sample will be taken to check for bladder infection, though this is unlikely to be found.

Other conditions that could be mistaken for NSU include not only cystitis (i.e. inflammation of the bladder lining) but also chronic inflammation of the prostate or balanitis (inflammation of the head of the penis and foreskin, with symptoms of an itchy and painful penis, which could be due to various things – tight foreskin, chemical irritation, infection with organisms).

What's the treatment?

NSU usually clears up with a course of antibiotics. The choice of drug depends on what's causing the problem, though this may not be known, as we've seen. The recommended treatment of first choice is doxycycline; usually 100mg twice a day for seven days, or a single 1g dose of azithromycin, or other antibiotics such as erythromycin or Deteclo, which are good at getting rid of NSU.

You should be checked a couple of weeks after treatment has finished so that another urethral smear can be done to see if you're cured or whether further treatment is needed.

During treatment

The urethra needs time to heal so don't have sex until *all* of the following has happened: your symptoms have gone; treatment has been completed and you've been given the all clear; and your partner has been treated – otherwise you could get reinfected.

Symptoms sometimes hang on for a bit even though the infection has gone so allow time for the urethra to get back to normal. Cut out alcohol or restrict how much you drink during treatment, as alcohol can irritate the urethra sometimes.

NSU that keeps coming back

If you keep getting problems you may need further drug treatments like erythromycin which is often given together with metronidazole. If you have complications like inflammation of the prostate other drug treatments may be used.

Partners

It's very important that your partner is tested and treated even if they have no symptoms. Women often have none, but you could be getting some infection from your female partner that is responsible for your problems and you could get reinfected if she isn't treated. Also, if women do have some untreated infection (e.g. gonorrhoea) they may be at risk of developing serious complications, such as pelvic inflammatory disease. If your urethral problems are caused by chlamydia, your female partner should automatically be treated for chlamydia even if the infection isn't detected in her – to play safe.

Prevention

Practise safer sex.

Pubic lice

What are they?

Pubic lice are tiny parasitic insects that live on the body in coarse body hair (e.g. pubic hair, underarm hair, hairy legs, abdomen and chest). Sometimes they're called 'crabs' because they look a bit like crabs under the microscope.

How do you get them?

Through close body contact, usually sexual though it may also be possible to get them by sharing sheets and towels. They travel by crawling from hair to hair; they don't fly or jump. They're not the same as head lice, which don't cause problems in the pubic area.

What are the symptoms?

Symptoms, which are the result of an allergy to the lice, include itching. Signs of pubic lice are black powder in your underwear from their droppings; brown eggs (nits) on pubic or other hair, sometimes you may see the lice on your skin. You may get symptoms straightaway or one or two weeks after exposure to the lice. If you have lice for a long time, the itching may stop as you become used to them.

How are they diagnosed?

A doctor examines you and inspects the pubic lice under a microscope to confirm the diagnosis.

What's the treatment?

It's easy to get rid of pubic lice using a special shampoo or lotion applied to the body. It's important to wash your clothes and bedding in hot water, 60°C, to avoid reinfection. Once treatment is finished, have a check-up to make sure you're clear of the lice. Even though treatment is successful, you may feel itchy for a few more weeks afterwards so ask your doctor whether you can have antihistamine treatment for this.

Various treatments are available over the counter from the pharmacy but it's best to see your doctor to make sure of a correct diagnosis.

What if you're pregnant?

Make sure the doctor or pharmacist knows, as this will affect the choice of treatment.

Partners

To avoid passing the lice on, don't have sexual contact until you've been successfully treated. Get your partner to be checked and treated if necessary.

Scabies

What is it?

Scabies is a skin infestation caused by the mite, *Sarcoptes scabiei*, when the female mites burrow into the skin and lay eggs. It's passed on through close physical contact with someone, which can include sexual contact. The mites die after 72 hours if they're kept away from their human host. Scabies is highly contagious and quite common.

What are the symptoms?

- Symptoms are an allergic reaction to the mites. A rash or tiny spots appear, usually a couple of weeks after you're infected as the body reacts to the mites. Tiny, grey, scaly swellings develop, usually between the fingers, on the top of your wrists and elbows, around the genitals, in the armpits, underneath the buttocks, abdomen and breasts, especially around the nipples in women. In adults, the palms, soles of the feet, neck, face and scalp aren't usually affected.

- The swellings can cause intense irritation, particularly at night or after a hot bath or shower.

Are there any complications?

None normally though occasionally you may develop a bacterial infection, in which case you may need antibiotic treatment.

How is it diagnosed?

By taking a medical history and doing a physical examination. (If you're taking steroids for asthma or have applied a steroid cream to the rash it may be harder to see the rash, because steroids suppress the immune system and scabies symptoms are a result of the body's immune response to the mites.) A skinflake from one of the spots is examined under a microscope to look for the mite or its droppings.

What's the treatment?

Special skin lotions containing malathion and permethrin are used, normally applied to the body from the neck down and washed off after 12 hours. If this doesn't work, there's a new tablet treatment called Ivermectin, which may be prescribed in addition to a lotion.

Clothing and bedding should be washed at a high temperature, above 60°C. Itching may continue for a couple of weeks after treatment even though the mites have been killed, so ask your doctor for antihistamine treatment to stop the itching.

Pregnancy

Make sure your doctor knows you're pregnant as this will affect treatment.

Partners

Sexual partners should be treated and all members of your household. You shouldn't have sex until you've finished treatment and are clear of the mites.

Syphilis

What is it and how common is it?

Syphilis is potentially a very serious infection caused by the bacterium. *Treponema pallidum*, a spirochaete (spiral shaped bacterium), which penetrates broken skin or mucous membranes (soft, pink, skin-like layer that lines various places in the body, such as the mouth) in the genitals, anus or mouth during sex. Ultimately it affects the whole body. It's not a common infection in the UK nowadays but there was a 55 per cent increase between 1999 and 2000, with just over 300 cases diagnosed. It's mainly sexually transmitted and mostly affects gay men, with the increase in cases in 2000 being mainly among homosexuals.

What are the symptoms?

Symptoms are the same in men and women and may take up to three months to show after sexual contact with someone who is infected. Syphilis has several stages.

Primary stage

One or more painless sores (chancres), which you may not notice, appear where the bacteria entered the body, about 21 days later on average, though the range is about 10 to 90 days. A sore is a painless ulcer, less than 1cm across, which can occur anywhere (e.g. the anus, mouth or urethra and in women on the lips of the vagina, the clitoris and the cervix and in men on the penis and foreskin). The sores may take several weeks to heal. The disease is highly infectious at this stage.

Secondary stage

Left untreated this stage occurs about 6 to 12 weeks after the appearance of the sores. Symptoms include a rash, which isn't itchy, over the whole body or in patches that may recur over several months. Flat, warty-looking growths appear on the vulva in women and around the anus in both men and women. Flu-like illness, tiredness, loss of appetite, also swollen glands, patchy hair loss, white patches on the tongue or roof of the mouth are experienced. The disease is highly infectious at this stage.

Latent stage

The latent stage, during which the infected person seems to have no signs or symptoms of the disease, can last for a few years or indefinitely. If untreated at this point, the disease progresses to another phase. Syphilis isn't infectious at this stage.

Tertiary stage

This normally starts within 10 years of the original infection but could be three years from infection or as late as 25 years. However, it's very rare these days because most people are treated before syphilis gets to this point. The tertiary stage can result in very serious health problems, such as organ damage, heart and nervous system damage, and brain damage, called 'neurosyphilis'. The disease isn't infectious at this stage.

How is syphilis passed on?

Mainly through unprotected sex and also through kissing and other intimate bodily contact (e.g. touching the affected areas). Oral sex has been responsible for many of the cases of syphilis among gay men since 1999. At the primary and secondary stages, a pregnant woman can pass the infection to her baby, which may result in stillbirth or the baby being born with various health problems.

How is it diagnosed?

Tests include a blood sample to look at your immune responses to the bacteria – it may take up to three months after infection to show up as positive. Other tests include examining fluid from a sore under the microscope to look for the bacteria, a physical examination, an internal examination for women, a urine sample.

What's the treatment?

Treatment for syphilis will cure the infection during the first two stages, the primary and secondary ones. If treatment doesn't happen until the latent stage, the infection can be cured but any heart or nervous system damage that's already occurred may be irreversible.

The best treatment is penicillin, normally a two-week course (if you're allergic to penicillin, say so, and another type of drug will be used). Treatment can cause a short-lived reaction, which occurs shortly after treatment due to the rapid killing of the bacteria, and you may get symptoms such as fever, chills, aches and pains but this isn't normally too serious.

After treatment you need to be monitored for at least a year to see how you are.

What about sex?

You shouldn't have any sort of sex until you're clear of infection.

What about pregnancy?

As I said earlier, untreated syphilis can be passed from a mother to her baby and babies born with syphilis have lifelong health problems. Nowadays pregnant women are tested for syphilis and, if treatment is needed, penicillin can be safely used.

Partners

It's very important that all partners should be tested and treated for infection.

Prevention

Practise safer sex.

Trichomonas vaginalis

Trichomonas vaginalis (trichomoniasis) is caused by a tiny parasite, which produces an infection in the vagina, and in the urethra in men. In 1999, there were 6,406 cases reported at UK sexual health clinics.

How do you get it?

Almost always from sexual contact and from contact between the penis and vagina. It may be transmitted in lesbian sex – for instance, on a vibrator if an infected woman uses the toy on herself and then on her partner without cleaning the sex toy in between usages. But you can't get the infection from oral or anal sex as far as we know. It's theoretically possible that the parasite can live outside the body for several hours and be transmitted by non-sexual means (e.g. through shared towels), though this is thought to be extremely unlikely. Occasionally a pregnant woman may pass the infection to her baby during a vaginal delivery.

What are the symptoms?

Women

- A few women, around 5 per cent, have no symptoms.
- Symptoms may occur between 3 and 21 days after infection. Seventy per cent of women notice a change in vaginal discharge, which may increase, become thinner, frothy or yellow/green in colour and perhaps develop a musty, fish smell; you may also have soreness, inflammation and itching in and around the vagina, painful sex, pain and burning when you pee.

Men

There are often no symptoms but when they occur may include a discharge from the penis – this will be thin and white in colour and may stain underwear – and pain when urinating.

Are there any complications?

Complications are very rare; it's not usually a serious infection.

How is it diagnosed?

Sometimes it's discovered during a cervical smear because the cervix may have a strawberry look about it, which can be seen with the naked eye sometimes. Diagnosis involves doing a pelvic examination in women, and taking a swab from the discharge so that this can be examined under a microscope to look for evidence of the parasites. A urethral swab is taken from men.

What's the treatment?

The infection can be successfully treated with an antibiotic such as metronidazole, best taken as a pill, usually twice daily for five to seven days or alternatively in one large single dose. You shouldn't have alcohol with this drug as it'll make you very sick.

What about sex?

Don't have it until you're given the 'all clear'.

What about pregnancy?

Infected pregnant women may be more at risk of having an early labour. Babies can also be infected during a vaginal delivery, which can mean they get genital or lung infections so treatment is important. Drug treatment with metronidazole over five to seven days can usually be given at all stages in pregnancy.

Partners

Partners should be tested and treated even if they have no symptoms because they could be infected.

Prevention

Practise safer sex.

8

Where to Get More Information

Services

Association of Genito-Urinary Medicine website – www.agum. org.uk – is designed for sexual health practitioners, so the language is a bit technical, but the site has useful information.

British Liver Trust telephone – 01473 276326 – for leaflets on the hepatitis viruses. Website – www.britishlivertrust.org.uk

Brook Advisory Centres helpline – 0800 0185 023 – provides a free sex-advice service for young people.

Durex website – www.durex.co.uk

Family Planning Association helpline – 0845 310 1334.

Health Promotion England website – www.lovelife.com – has information on infections.

Herpes Viruses Association helpline – 020 7609 9061 – or send an SAE for information to 41 North Road, London N7 9DP.

London Lesbian and Gay Switchboard – 020 7837 7324.

Marie Stopes International website – www.likeitis.org.uk – has been developed for under-16-year-olds.

National Institute of Medical Herbalists – 01392 426022 – website – www.NIMH.org.uk

NHS Direct information and advice service – 0845 46 47.

Public Health Laboratory Service website – www.phls.co.uk – gives facts and figures on STIs.

Relate website – www.relate.org.uk – for help with relationship issues.

Sexual Health and National AIDS helpline (free) – 0800 567 123 – provides information on HIV and other sexually transmitted infections.

Sexware, FP Sales Ltd, Mail Order Dept, PO Box 833, Oxford OX4 5NT for condoms, etc.

Society of Sexual Health Advisers in Sexually Transmitted Diseases has a useful website – www.shastd.org.uk – which the public can use.

Terrence Higgins Trust helpline – 020 7242 1010 – provides information on HIV and AIDS.

Other

Holidays – before travelling abroad, get a copy of 'Your Passport to Sexual Health', about STIs and contraception. The leaflet is free, on sending an SAE to Marie Stopes International (Passport), 153–7 Cleveland Street, London W1T 6QW.

Men's health website – www.malehealth.co.uk

Books

Julia Cole, *Find the Love of Your Life*, Hodder & Stoughton, 2001. Written by a sex therapist.

Anne Edwards, Jackie Sherrard, Jonathan Zenilman, *Fast Facts: Sexually Transmitted Infections*, Health Press, 2001. Written for health professionals.

Lisa Marr, *Sexually Transmitted Diseases: A Physician Tells You What You Need to Know*, Johns Hopkins University Press, 1998. A guide to all infections written by a US doctor.

Index